BRINGING COMFORT
HOPE IN TIMES OF SUFFERING

Maryann P. Hobbie

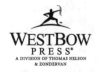

WESTBOW
PRESS®
A DIVISION OF THOMAS NELSON
& ZONDERVAN

WestBow Press books may be ordered through booksellers or by contacting:

WestBow Press
A Division of Thomas Nelson & Zondervan
1663 Liberty Drive
Bloomington, IN 47403
www.westbowpress.com
844-714-3454

Cover imagery by Maryann P. Hobbie. Initial design by Ellen Weisbord.

St. Joseph Edition of the New American Bible
Copyright 1970 by the Catholic Book Publishing Co., New York
Confraternity of Christian Doctrine, Washington D.C.

ISBN: 978-1-6642-3466-6 (sc)
ISBN: 978-1-6642-3467-3 (hc)
ISBN: 978-1-6642-3465-9 (e)

Library of Congress Control Number: 2021909819

Print information available on the last page.

WestBow Press rev. date: 6/4/2021

Dedicated to

Ewa Jessica Wolowicz

Because I promised...

With special thanks to

Every dear aide who treated me with dignity, respect and love
The Hobbie clan
The medical team that saved my life
My rehab hospital family
The parish community of Our Lady of the Magnificat
My Seton Hall University family
My Circle of Friends, Ian in the lead
Audrey, Kerry, Jody, Kelly, Dianne, Linda and Peg
Bob Jones
Julia Cameron for her morning pages
Brenda Forte and Sue Tepper, PTSD therapists extraordinaire
The Knights of Malta, especially the McLoughlins
For my grand baby, who kept me fighting
For my NJ Access Link bus drivers and friends
And most especially for True Blue,
My faithful, loving, kind and generous forester husband,
Richard S. Wolowicz

Spirit's words to me

Lourdes, France

My child, I have promised you a new direction and a new beginning. Indeed, I am healing you of maladies of the soul still unknown to you. You will write with a speed and lucidity unknown to you before, for I have created you, knit you in your mother's womb, yes, and have used my Mother to bring others to me. She understands you, child, She who is full of grace… Stay here with me child. Right here.

My child, indeed I am here with you, close to you, cleansing you. I've made space within you…I will reveal all that you need to know. Stay close to me. I will show you what to do.

CONTENTS

INTRODUCTION

This is not the book I had planned on writing. God had another idea.

So, yes, once I was a vent-dependent tetraplegic, C4-C7, incomplete, or as my friend says, "paralyzed from the neck down," and before that, I was dying in ICU. But the medical interventions of an outstandingly attentive medical team saved my life.

In my three-month blackout which marks the beginning of my hospitalization, I do remember this one thing. I told God: "God, I'm not ready to go home yet. I don't want to leave my husband, my daughter, my grandbaby, my Seton Hall students or my church kids. But if You want me to, I will."

And the voice answered: *I am not finished with you yet. I have work for you to do.*

And here, my friends, is some of the work. Many of the stories aren't easy to read, nor were they always easy to write, for there is much pain associated with them. During my eight month journey living in medical institutions which included a neuro ICU, a rehab and a nursing home... my entire life was changed.

Dramatically.

But the most important change is that it opened my heart to love.

If you ask the Spirit to lead you, Spirit will. Spirit knows the depth of your hurt, your fear, your anger and confusion. Cry out, just like the composers of the psalms or the prophet Jeremiah did and lay *all* of your burdens upon our Creator. Then turn these pages, find your prayer or a story that feeds your soul. Look for an angel that the Spirit will send.

Spirit will not leave you alone.

You are never alone.

Peace, my friend. Peace.

Spirit's words to me

My child, indeed I am getting you ready for a profound summer of concentration in writing from way deep down inside. My words are within. They will penetrate your consciousness. Put all else aside that you may hear my words, my precious one. It is all about me this summer, how you have been shaped and formed. Indeed the book will seem like new to you. My words will be a big part of it as they are of grace. Suffering souls will be touched, others will be strengthened. My fallen away friends will come nearer. My child, it is not for you to focus on end results, just write from the heart. Walk, run, be outdoors indeed, be on your mat so that you can breathe deeply and connect with me... it is up to you to listen. Rejoice indeed, my child; a new chapter has begun. Do not be diverted. Write for me, my child, write. Indeed I will show you where to start. Trust in me. Explore your new impulses. I am here, within you. Hear me. My Blessed Mother has assisted and will continue to assist you — knots have been untied and you have been bathed in my healing waters. Do not be diverted. Write for me and my children, write...

A TRIBUTE

It is a daunting task. To adequately pay homage to each of the women who cared for me over the seasons of my hospitalization would take, at the least, another book.

And gentlemen? I haven't forgotten your role in my healing and to each one of you I am forever grateful.

But for now, I want to focus on the ladies.

There are so many stories I could write about your strengths and giftedness that graced my life throughout the times of my most dire need. Today, I no longer separate my physicality from my spirituality, my soul's well-being from that of my physical body. Because of that, I know now that you fed my soul as you cared for, tended to and challenged my broken body. Each of you served as *living messengers* of grace and dignity, nurturance and hope, light and life, when I needed those things the most to survive and eventually, to thrive. To name each of you would be an impossible task and to highlight only a few of you would do a great disservice to the others that remain anonymous or hidden in the shadows of my memory.

So instead, please accept my letter of love. You know you will always have a place deep in my heart. I wanted to let each and every one of you know how grateful I am to you and forever will be. Your care and concern has enabled me to be the woman I am today, here to serve however God chooses.

My memory is erased for three months of my life, so I'll have to be content with sending one big sweeping 'thank you' to all those women who cared for me and whose amazing skills helped keep me here on this earth during that time. I may not remember you, but I thank you with every ounce of my strong, beating heart, my every breath taken without the assistance of any machine.

And when I finally did awaken, dazed and confused, it did not take long for the fog to clear enough for me to realize just how many special women were caring for me.

For the women who teamed up to turn me in the beginning: I am told that I cried from the pain whenever anyone touched me, when your gentle hands turned me, cleaned me, changed me. Although I don't remember those earliest days, I know you tried to comfort me with your always compassionate presence. Adept in your professionalism, you helped me in my time of greatest need...and for that, I thank you.

For my doctor, with her wonderful laughter: I trusted in you and relied upon you with literally every fiber of my being.

For the nurses (male and female): I depended upon you every morning as I started a new day, through every afternoon and then every evening that so often became yet another long, taxing and exacting night. You taught me about my meds, my feedings and you taught me to hope. Always.

For the myriad of therapists and all their talents: Each one of you encouraged me, challenged me, taught me. You wouldn't let me say, "I can't." You insisted, subtly, overtly, that my life was still valuable and showed me how to view things differently. You revolutionized my thinking. You never allowed me to condemn myself to the self-made prison of comparing my present skill set with what I could do before the injury. Instead, you taught me to celebrate every victory. *"Live in the present."* It wasn't a mantra; it's what you showed me, modeled for me, lived for me. Go team!

For that really tall lady in the business suit: you first got my attention when you walked through the therapy gym. You carried yourself regally, yet, discreetly. I knew you were a woman of honor, integrity and prayer, respected and revered by so many. Thank you for the encouragement and inspiration you always were to me.

And for the aides, forever my dearest treasures: No amount of stories could ever be told that would fully encapsulate the amount of love you gave me. Through your never-ending belief in me, your patience and understanding and yes, your gentleness and kindness, you helped to heal my broken heart. You treated me with dignity and respect...always. You lifted me up; you were kind to me. I know that many of you carried heavy burdens with you from home; I learned to read it in your face, see it in your eyes or perhaps feel a slight change in your energy, your mood. But somehow, you managed to put those burdens aside when you entered my room. You gave your heart and full attention to me, a mere infant sometimes, in my long and skinny broken body.

You gave me hope.

With all my heart, my ladies, I thank you.

Bless you, bless you, bless you.

Spirit's words to me

I am sending you out on a mission. Walk in my love, CLAIM my victory over darkness and evil, for you have been transformed in me. You no longer have to cower in a corner, child. You are my beloved creation, my grace has transformed you… Recognize and claim my sovereignty. My words will continue to come to you. I will make my way abundantly clear. No more cowering, child, in the fear of lies - of old beliefs that do not suit you. I have risen and you have risen with me. Yes child, you were headed toward the grave, but you asked me and I answered you. My child, my child, I am not finished with you. I have work for you to do.

BEGINNINGS

The summer of 2013 had promised to be a spectacular one. Old dreams were about to be manifested, some hopes restored. Indeed, I was embarking on a journey of transformation and healing, but not at all in the way I had envisioned it.

Almost thirty years prior to this, while an administrator at Georgian Court College, I had the privilege of chaperoning some of our students for an art tour of Rome. It was love at first sight. I was infatuated with the sculptures and the ancient buildings and was completely captivated by every square inch of the Vatican Museum. After my trip, I included at least one class about renaissance art in each of my college courses. I would lug in a huge pile of my own heavy art books for the students to review. Eurocentric, perhaps, but I believed that whatever the student's major, an education was not complete without exposure to the Sistine Chapel! As often as I could, I urged undergraduates to travel and study abroad, enthusiastically encouraging them to explore the world and all of its astounding beauty. Throughout the years, the desire to return to feast my eyes and soul on Rome's artistic treasures burned deeply inside of my heart.

Finally, that desire came to its fruition. One morning, I received an email that advertised a Seton Hall University faculty and staff retreat in Rome, aptly named "A Journey of Transformation." The retreat was sponsored by the Center for Catholic Studies and subsidized by their generous donors. Both the Center and the retreat were directed by our beloved Msgr. Richard Liddy, whose scholarship and gentle soul have touched so many members of the Seton Hall community, student, staff and faculty alike.

It was an offer I couldn't refuse.

Initially, I felt ecstatic. But then, I reasoned, it would be unfair to spend that money on myself. More importantly, our new grandbaby would only be a few months old. She and her teenaged college freshman mom would need me at home to help them.

"Oh, no," my best friend and running companion of almost fifteen years chided me. "You've been talking about going back to Rome for years! The baby and your daughter will be fine. And if you try to back out," she paused for emphasis here, "I will personally drive you to the airport and put you on the plane!"

And, so, off to Rome I went.

I would never tire of the beauty that awaited me. Our seven days were woven through with times for learning and reflection. We toured beautiful churches and went for a walk with a monk reading St. Augustine's *Confessions* out loud in his lovely lilting brogue. We visited the hauntingly austere residence and church of St Ignatius Loyola, the founder of the Jesuits. Each day we heard fascinating lectures by a broad range of scholars. The art historian Elizabeth Lev gave us the tour of a lifetime for two brief days.

And then, there was my birthday. My mother had once told me that when she was coming down the stairs of our old house to leave for the hospital to give birth to me, she heard the Magnificat chiming from our local parish church of Saint John the Evangelist. I'd like to think that someday my soul could magnify the Lord like Mary's did. Thinking back upon my life, I knew that I wasn't quite there yet, but perhaps this was a start. Here I was in Rome, celebrating the day of my birth, gathering with the crowds in St. Peter's Square to await the arrival of the Pope.

As an avid photographer, I was already reeling from the beauty of the buildings, edifices, nooks and crannies all about me in the ancient city of Rome. Now, behind the anonymity of my camera, I began to study the faces of the people anxiously awaiting the Pope's arrival. No one gave any thought to me as my long lens captured the emotional drama playing out upon their faces. Intuitively, I knew that their expressions would tell me the moment they spotted their beloved new Pope Francis. But, when that moment came, I beheld something so powerful that it was beyond my immediate comprehension. On every face my lens could capture, all tension had melted into joy. Their faces literally glowed with a sudden new light, a tangible warmth, an exuberance.

I had witnessed a transformation.

They were transformed...*but I was not.* I felt my smallness, my separateness, my limitedness. In the rawness of the moment, I was laid bare:

jaded, jagged, the worn edges of lassitude and disappointment corroding my heart. I felt distant and locked away inside myself.

Sometimes, I just hated being me.

But, no matter; I was well-practiced in putting on a show for the world. Swallowing those feelings back down as quickly as they came up, I denied them any further power over me. Instead, I invited the joy and the wonder of being in Rome to envelop my spirit.

Excitement renewed, I gathered with our group for the next stop on our agenda: the Vatican Museum. As we waited on the steps for our tour guide, I was already feeling like a little kid on Christmas Eve! Then, a fellow retreat member extended to me an invitation beyond my wildest dreams. She invited me to teach back home in Seton Hall University's Catholic Studies Program.

Unbeknownst to anyone but my dear Msgr. Liddy, I had been carrying a secret, a source of great shame inside of me. While working on my doctorate, I'd had the opportunity to teach for several years in a neighboring university. College teaching had always been a passion for me and my classes were well-received. I had been looking forward to earning my degree, so that I could continue to open minds in my classrooms and have the freedom to teach in the area of my specialties. However, my doctoral studies were abruptly terminated upon the ill-fated conclusion of my comprehensive exams. My then-undiagnosed learning disability had thwarted me once again.

Thankfully, I was still able to hold a teaching position as an adjunct instructor at my beloved Seton Hall. I was enthralled with every aspect of their new Catholic Studies program, which explored the magnificent contributions of thought and culture in the Catholic intellectual tradition. I knew, though, that without my doctorate in hand, I would remain painfully excluded from the inner sanctum of academia. That is, until that moment when I received the invitation on the steps of the Vatican Museum.

As we made our way into the museum, my heart was bursting with joy. I felt suddenly redeemed (at least momentarily) from the burdens I'd carried on my shoulders since grad school: the weight of shame, of failure, of academic disgrace. Incredulous questioning began inside my head: *Was this really happening to me? Teach?! Seton Hall had invited me to teach in their Catholic Studies Program??*

Senses heightened, I moved with the group into the cool quiet of the vast museum halls. Soon, we were standing in the hushed and reverent stillness created by the overpowering beauty of Michelangelo's *Pietà*. My mind could not process the thought of how a twenty-four-year-old artist could even conceive of this living memorial. My breath caught as I gazed upon Mary holding the figure of her Son draped lifeless across her lap; I could feel the white marble breathing her pain. Mesmerized, I stood staring at her face. Then, my eyes, ever so slowly moved down to her Son. I followed the long, lean lines of His body, which conveyed a strong sense of a life filled with effortless movement, flowing with grace and dignity. But now, in death, His once strong right arm hung dangling, powerless, toward the floor. My heart tore in anguish as my own memories rose to the surface. Oh, the ache that had consumed my whole being when I saw my precious daughter, a mere ten years old, emerge yet again from one of many childhood surgeries. As the nurse was asking permission to pump morphine into that tiny body, I felt powerless over my own child, powerless to help her pain. That had been bad enough, but this...? I couldn't even begin to imagine the horror of holding the lifeless body of my own child.

As if in a trance, I found it difficult to pull away; I did not want to leave this Mother and her Son. Finally I turned, my heart heavy, forcing myself to separate from their presence. I walked away, grieving and profoundly touched.

As the tour continued, we wound our way through the halls and gardens of the museum. The magnificence, the beauty, the grandeur of the art - the sculptures, the paintings - continued to overwhelm me. I was entranced by each new breathtaking sight, my being consumed. By the time we approached the end of our tour, my heart and soul were drenched with wonder.

Our final destination of the day was the one I most eagerly anticipated: the Sistine Chapel. The moment I stepped through the doorway, I gasped, frozen, in utter shock and awe. When I had been here thirty years ago, time had worn down the paintings to dull and grey. Since then, artists had been called in to painstakingly restore them. Now, the five-hundred-year-old masterpieces on the ceilings and walls pulsed with life, vigor and invitation. Story after story gloriously unfurled their powerful tales, lessons and majesty.

As the colors of the transformed frescoes seared through to my soul, a question boldly formed in my mind: *Could I, too, be restored?* After all, this was my birthday, a day of blessings and new beginnings. So much was beginning to stir deep down inside of me. Old feelings and fears were battling, trying to capture me, trap me, reminding me that I would probably fail, as I had always failed before. Feeling the power of the dissonance rising within my spirit, I struggled to push those fears back down, back to where all of my other fears lived. Determined not to let them drown me, I staunchly refused to give them any air time or to allow them to ruin my new beginnings.

Excited and invigorated by the retreat and all of its gifts, I returned home to my waiting family (husband, daughter and three month old grandbaby)...and to my new running group! Having left marathons and racing behind me, I had, with the exception of an occasional jog with my friend, been running alone on trails and roads for years. But while on the faculty retreat in Rome, I met a colleague who just happened to live in the town next to mine. She invited me to join her group of nine women, each of whom were committed to various running goals and competitions throughout the summer and fall.

On my first few runs with the group, I was chagrined by my lack of speed. Self-conscious, but resolute, I stayed at the back of the pack. There, I could listen intently to all of the wonderful conversations without necessarily joining in. Within a few weeks of training, though, my body had caught up with my ambition. Soon, I, too, was holding conversations while running and mulling over new opportunities to compete again.

Friday, 26 July marked my best run of the summer...and the beginning of my worst nightmare. That night, we had to put my soulmate, our beloved standard poodle, Prancer Sequoia Mozart, to sleep.

My heart broke – and in my sleep, my body broke, too.

My spectacular summer was no more.

I woke up in the morning and couldn't swallow. My daughter tried to help me with breakfast. I remember that much, but then...? My memory fades until mid-October, when I regained full conscious awareness to find a trach in my throat, a feeding tube in my stomach, a myriad of IV's snaking about my arms and my tall, strong runner's body paralyzed from the neck down. My official diagnosis: *tetraplegic, C4- C7, incomplete.*

Of the prior weeks and months, I remember very little. I am told that my life on this planet appeared to be nearing its end. I am absolutely convinced that during this time, the constant visits and fervent prayers of my distraught and anxious family, friends, university and parish community managed to keep me here on this earth.

Through the haziness, I do remember saying a prayer.

"God, I'm not ready to go home yet. I do not want to leave my husband, my daughter, my grandbaby, my youth ministry kids at church, or my Seton Hall students. But if that is what You want, You can take me."

And the voice answered: *I am not finished with you yet. I have work for you to do.*

And here is some of that work. Within the covers of this book may you find a story or a prayer or two that resonates within you, that perhaps brings you some comfort. May the God who helped me write this book bring you hope and comfort, even in the midst of your feelings of anger, abandonment and aloneness. Know that I was once there, too, battling with agony and anguish that threatened to drown me at every turn. And, dear reader, please know that those feelings do *not* have to overcome you, those feelings do *not* have to win! Today my vision is different, my being transformed through the many lessons learned through those harrowing times. May your present difficulties, painful as they may be, bring transformation to you as well. It may take time, but my hope is that your heart will heal and reveal new ways of being in the world.

But, most of all, may you discover the love of the one who created you and brought you into this world. May you discover on your journey what I discovered on mine:

You are loved.

You are never alone.

God is with you.

And so am I.

May you find hope.

Spirit's words to me

...Search your notebooks for my words. Write them up. They will indeed supply the structure you are searching for. My way will be made clear. My words will flow. Just calling me to guide you and we will move swiftly and steadily through – I have been renewing your heart since you gave it to me in Lent – and now the Easter season is drawing to a close and you can celebrate your life anew. The presence of My Counselor, your Advocate will lead you strong and true. Step up and into the light my child. You have bathed in my waters at Lourdes, you have been renewed. You needn't hold back. Celebrate my love. Go as deep as you can my child, go deep. I will not let go of you. I heal the pain child - of others, of my own – I heal their pain. Readers will find comfort as I renew my presence through your story of hope and connection, passion and suffering. Indeed, brokenness may be the human condition, healing is the divine. Come to me all you who labor and are heavy with burdens and I will give you rest. Come my child, write so my children can be fed. Write.

TREES (BROKEN)

They stood in a stand: stark white trees, empty of leaves, stretching their winter limbs up to the leaden, grey November sky.

This was my first time out of the hospital in four months. We were on our way to my sister's house to celebrate a family Thanksgiving, a miracle day. My eyes were fixated, my breath caught, on what I was seeing to the right of the highway. Dozens and dozens of trees stood white, pure white in my memory, naked of their summer leaves, stretching, stretching up to the late fall sky.

But what really captured my attention was that in every single tree there laid a broken limb. Each was still uplifted, nestled sideways, comforted and secure in the outstretched arms of their intact neighbors.

The vision is seared into my brain.

We drove past that stand of trees, but the metaphors that scene represented stayed way down deep inside me. Two years later, while I trained to become a chaplain, the metaphors emerged again and evolved as poems in my *Broken* series, arising phoenix-like, amongst the darkness and brokenness all around me. I began to use those images as gathering-prayer poems on class days for my fellow student chaplains. Through those poems, I would speak to my classmates about what I saw that day and the meaning it held for me:

Beautiful broken limbs, cradled in the arms of their surrounding trees. Even broken and suspended, these limbs were just as important to their forest community as when they were fully attached to the trunk of their tree. It matters not to their Maker that they were broken. They had just changed appearances.

They were still important.

Like that stand of trees, God has placed us here on this earth together. We can lean on each other, support each other, lift each other up when we have fallen down. We can learn to be community. Yes, even though we come from a myriad of backgrounds, I still believe that we are not that much different from each other. Each one of us is unique, singularly shaped by life's gifts, its offerings, its challenges and sufferings, forming us into individuals seemingly separate and distinct. But internally, we have all been wounded. Somewhere, we have all experienced brokenness.

Some of us wear our brokenness on the outside. We came into the world that way, or maybe we were broken later in life. No matter how we live our brokenness, we are one.

Like me, so many of my friends have broken bodies. Each one of us are born with gifts and talents that have vital parts to play in this universe. We yearn to use them.

The appearance of our bodies sometimes makes others feel uncomfortable and awkward around us. We can sense that.

Maybe we don't move graciously, maybe we stutter our words. So did Moses. God still used him for His purpose. He sent Moses' brother Aaron to help him out.

May we learn not to dismiss each other. Our time together on this grand earth is very short; we all need each other.

Stay open, my friends. Stay open to the gift and depth of brokenness.

Spirit's words to me

...Relax in my love, in my grace, in the splendor of my glorious rains and sunshine, my summer flowers holding my beauty. I am holding you my child. Your broken heart held Della so close to you. I know my child. I know your heartache. The words are right here, my child, the words are right here. Carry your notebook and your pen and your iPad, too—and just listen, listen and be still. The words will come unbidden as I shower my grace on you, my conduit of peace, my vessel of love. Presence and word, writing I reveal myself through you. Stay open, pray for grace. I take great joy in you as you fill the well, waking up to the joy of my creation around you... My child you are my beloved, my precious one... Be still. Breathe. Know that I am with you. Rejoice. Rejoice. You are my Easter triumph my child, my Advent awakened—as you waited you turned to me. I sent you a dear friend to start your writing journey. She prays for you child—many do—yes, indeed, I have much work for you to do. Just ask to be in my presence—all the rest will come.

ALMOST HOME - TILT TABLE

And then there was the time I almost went home.

Almost.

It happened in my early days in the therapy gym at rehab. I was working with my physical therapist doing my least favorite physical therapy activity: *the tilt table*. The table was quite a simple construction. It was a black, shiny 4-foot-wide by 8 foot long cushioned board with a footrest on one end. When a patient was strapped onto it, the physical therapist would press a switch that operated the quiet, yet eerie sounding motor located underneath. Then in gradual intervals, the therapist could tilt the table up, safely and progressively transitioning the patient to an upright position.

I hated it.

I did not feel safe on that table. I hated the idea of being separated from the ground and removed from my peers there. I wanted to be on the mats or in my chair at ground level with my friends. I'd always felt as if my fellow patients and I were like a giant amoeba. We throbbed as one with our movements and with our breaths, occasionally assisted with trachs and vents. We were all part of one another. Like mine, their bodies had been suddenly and unexpectedly mutilated before we were admitted, some by injury, some by disease. They understood. We were a tribe. Their presence, ground level, made me feel safe.

I also hated the idea of being removed from the security of my wheelchair and being suspended on the tilt table. Truthfully, I was petrified, but too cool to show it, or for that matter, to really admit it to myself. I loved being grounded on the earth; in fact I need the feel of the earth beneath my feet. It was bad enough that I could no longer walk on it. Already reeling from the disorientation caused by my paralysis, I felt that being hoisted into the air took away even more of my very thin semblance of security. After all, I barely tolerated being moved through the air on a kiddie Ferris wheel!

My physical therapist and an assistant would transfer me from the wheelchair to the Hoyer lift and finally, to the tilt table. It was no easy feat, but they did it with fluidity and grace. She would then ease me onto my back, maneuvering my lifeless body in her usual professional, proficient, loving manner, all the while explaining to me what was going to happen. There I would be strapped down, both across my torso and across my legs. I don't even remember feeling the pressure of the straps, but it was probably more the implication of the act that bothered me the most. If you tie someone down, they can't escape. They must be a danger to themselves or to others.

Powerless.

I hated feeling powerless. I felt like it was always being rubbed in my face: my powerlessness, no...my *helplessness*. I just couldn't help the feeling. It was coming from the droning of damning lies constantly looping in my head, the ones that cycled through their insulting condemnations that told me *I am never going to be good enough...I'm stupid...I'm a loser.* Every movement that I yearned to make, every task I wanted to jump up and do—simple ones, like lifting up an arm, bending over to tie my shoes, brushing my teeth, or opening a book and leafing through it to find a favorite passage—all of those desires mocked me. My body did not work for me anymore. It was merely a shell that housed my soul and spirit. Yes, my worn and bruised spirit now resided inside this cumbersome, lumbersome body.

Once I was securely fastened to the tilt table and the tilting initiated, my physical therapist would come and see how I was doing. At certain time intervals (was it five minutes or was it twenty?), she would check on me to see how I was feeling, checking to see if I was getting nauseated and other quick questions assessing my feelings of well-being and stamina. Then, she would check my blood pressure. If my body was not protesting she would carefully tilt the table even higher. Nausea was my incessant companion, as was the underlying terror that vomiting would cause me to choke. And although I could dimly "sense" a rolling throughout my belly, the rest of my sensations were dulled, if not absent. And so, I lived in constant fear that I might defecate at any moment...and not know about it.

My body was truly out of my control. Sometimes, it was mortifying.

Oh, how I hated it.

After I was strapped down and surreally suspended in the air, I would warily watch over all my fellow spinal cord injury friends in various phases of their gym activities. On this one particular afternoon, I spotted my latest roommate pedaling a stationary bike machine. She was sitting very low to the ground, her eyes closed, a small, serene smile on her beatific face.

I knew what she was doing. She had told me that each time she went into the gym, she would start singing psalms to herself. And there she was, in worship and praise, oblivious to all around her.

My physical therapist interrupted me.

"Let's try this Pandora today."

I didn't know what she was talking about. *Pandora…? Like, from Greek mythology?* A cell phone with earbuds appeared in my physical therapist's hands and she said that they had been mine! Not having communicated with the outside world in many months, I stared at them, feeling like she was holding an artifact from an ancient site, something from a different planet.

In answer to my quizzical look, she replied, "We asked your husband to bring these in, remember?"

I didn't.

It mattered not.

"I know you hate the tilt table, so why don't you try listening to some Pandora to distract you?"

"Sure," I replied, rather reluctantly. "Yes, you go ahead if you want."

She proceeded to slide the phone somewhere inside one of the straps and deftly put an earbud in each ear.

Strange. It was so incredibly strange to hear music while I was floating in the air, strapped down to my tilted gurney table. I felt weird and pretty creeped out. Over the past few weeks at rehab, I had grown to love and listen for Broadway Bill, the disc jockey who came on the radio in the afternoons at three o'clock. The music he played blasted through those speakers in the therapy gym and revved everybody up. His voice was soothing. He reminded me I wasn't alone.

But not now on the tilt table. With my earbuds anchored in, I couldn't hear Broadway Bill over the gym speakers. Instead, I was hearing music that I hadn't heard since my now 19-year-old daughter was small. I didn't know what was happening.

It was Alison Krauss singing about Jesus.

And then I saw...You.

I was in the therapy gym...right? But not really. All of a sudden, I was walking down this sunny beautiful road made of rich, terra cotta colored soil, majestic pine trees reaching to the skies on both sides of me. The path was wide and the day was clear and beckoning.

I was *walking*.

And I felt You behind me, my sweet, sweet, dear Jesus. I could see You behind me without turning my head. I was so peaceful and happy with You. I felt no fear. Your hands, like strong feathers, pressed up against my shoulders and kept me upright. And then I tried to lean back into You. You smiled, but You would not let me leave this earth.

You reminded me that I couldn't go home to You just yet. You reminded me – without speaking – that I still had work You wanted me to do for You.

I felt dejected, devastated, lost. I felt so physically close to You, my entire being saturated with a complete peace that surged through me, suffused in sudden understanding of the absence of suffering, about to go to my real home...

...and You said no. You were not ready for me.

The sadness that filled me was overwhelming.

And then...I was back in the gym again. Somehow, I was thrust back into the reality of being on the tilt table and where I really was. My physical therapist came by to check on me and saw nothing out of the ordinary. In the span of a few short moments, I completely forgot about Your visit.

A few days later when I returned to my room after therapy, there were a few get well cards waiting for me on my bed. When an aide came in to help get me ready, I asked her if she would be so kind as to open my mail and hold up the cards for me to read. I hated taking extra time from her. I knew she was busy and had many patients to shower, change or get ready for bed, so I felt my request was too self-indulgent. I hated asking anybody to go out of their way for me, ever.

But she was always so kind.

"Of course!" she quietly said and took a few steps over to my bedside. She opened and held the first card for me so I could read it. I remember how that card touched me deeply. I loved the fact that someone, anyone, had gone out of their way to encourage me, send prayers and well wishes. Oh, how I longed to hug and be held by my friends and communities in the outside world! Each and every card that was sent to me brought such comfort to my aching heart.

Not wanting to delay my dear aide any longer, I asked her to open my second card of the day. It was from someone at my beloved church, the community whose closeness I especially missed. The card was quite elaborate, a little booklet of pictures and prayers. My aide patiently turned the pages for me, allowing my eyes to slowly scan the illustrations and prayers. Suddenly, I gasped. There, on the page before me, was a picture of...You!

You. Somebody had painted the exact image of You as You had come to me in the gym; only they had put gold around Your robe.

I was speechless. Instantly, I was pulled back into the cocoon of Your love, so intimate, so blissfully engulfing and engaging as it was the other day. Since then, I had remained aware of your love but in a more remote, generalized sense of everyday knowing, so unlike and distinct from the warmth and feeling of overwhelming joy, peace and protection that You had graced me with on that beautiful tree-lined road deep in the forest of my vision.

It was You.

You.

It still makes me sad, thinking about that terrible aloneness...and the weight of those daily struggles to merely survive in my newly amended life. But it's comforting to remember those cards and to recall the love and support of the friends who uplifted me. Most significantly, it's comforting to remember Your visit.

You came to me in the gym and You made it a holy place. If You came to me, I know You come to others. It is You who created our hearts and souls, You who loves us as Your children. It is You who always senses our hidden pains, our anguish. It is You who heals our broken hearts, who tends to our brokenness of body, mind and spirit.

And yes, it is You who guides the hands, hearts and skills of each member of the spinal cord therapy gym team. Through them, You convert moments of pain and suffering into moments of grace. Barely discernible grace.

Through them, You loved me. Through them, You strengthened me.

Bless my silently singing roommate for being such a good example to me. Bless all the ones who fear the tilt table or any other physical or emotional challenges in the gym.

Divine Creator, You go anywhere. You have no barriers.

Bless the weary and the skeptical ones in the physical therapy gyms today. Bless the therapists and inspire them to do the right thing. Help them to know how important they are in their special work. They are the life-lines for so many.

Dear Lord, lift their burdens.

And bless the aides who assist them. They are the ones who move tons of material, cushions and apparatus, readying the mats for patients, cheering up and encouraging patients, or staying with them when they cry.

So much pain and hurt in the therapy gym, so much in each long day.

Give Your patients, therapists and aides endurance, Lord. Give them Your grace.

And bless their specially trained therapy dogs as well. These beautiful animals brought me moments of peace, of connection, when my soul was distraught. I had never even grieved for my dog, my soul mate, that precious, loving creature we had to put to sleep without warning the night before this whole nightmare began.

Tilt tables as conduits of Grace.

You didn't take me home that day Lord, and I wasn't happy that You left me.

But You didn't leave me.

Thank You, sweet Jesus.

Thank You.

Spirit's words to me

My child, indeed I have set you on a new path. Fulfillment is in union with me. Stay close to me, turn to me—I will give you words, direction and rest. Enjoy the life I have given you. See the abundance surrounding you. The words are right here. I will give you clear direction for my people are hurting, floundering. Say yes to me child. Rejoice in the birdsong—there will be more. Rejoice in my flowers, in my friends I send to you, young women and men, looking for me as they make their way in the world. They don't know how to find me child. Many don't want their parent's church and don't think they need me to 'make it' in this world. Ah, my child, they have no idea how much love I have for them, mercy in abundance. Keep saying yes child, let me alter your schedule where needed—breathe in me, breathe. Indeed, you get discontented with me. The homily did not celebrate my Pentecost—my reigning down of the Holy Spirit – can you do that for me? Celebrate the Holy Spirit in all her gifts this summer. She is here – Wisdom, Sophia – to guide you and make you strong, indeed, that was one of the ways you found me—your first mass in the [Seton Hall] chapel with Rich, October 1986—in the bulletin designed with Paul's scripture - the Spirit God has given us is no cowardly spirit, but one that is STRONG, LOVING and WISE - and that, my child, is who I have called you to be—STRONG, LOVING and WISE. You have met death and adversity – and you have found me... and you went through the adversity turning to me as best you could—and I heard the prayers that surrounded you. Many angels were sent your way. A fortress of prayers surrounded you – and I sent my people to support you. We became friends, my child, we became friends. And little by little your heart has opened and you are gaining a NEW vision, a NEW way of seeing things—from and through the heart my child—not just what is on the surface. I am here to feed you child, the Mother Pelican, the all–seeing, all-knowing Creator God—I am here, within, loving you... oh my sweet, sweet daughter enjoy this recovered life, this renewed life, this new walking life. My graces abound—do not separate yourself from me—your life BREATH.

WEEKENDS

This is the line of demarcation: Friday afternoon.
All therapy ends at four.
I wheel myself out of the rehab cocoon
of kindness and energy and support and challenge,
and into the cloying vortex
of loneliness.

The emptiness falls on me like a weight.
My web of support…
vanished.

I am alone.

I don't belong anywhere.

I'm not going away for the weekend to a wedding,
or traveling to meet some college friends
like many of the therapists
who still had a life.

I am going to my room.

To wait.

To be in the hurt and pain of being stripped of all I was before:
mom, wife, new grandma,
youth minister, college professor.

Now? I am nothing.

I am suspended from my life,
from all of my former identities.

During the weekdays, I rise to each therapy challenge,
following directions to move an arm, a limb,
anything I'm told.

And during the weekend—all that energy?
Gone.

It's an unbearable sensation, my awful feeling of emptiness.
It catches up with me at night.

But that's another story.

Weekends are enough.

They crush me with their weight.
My ghosts and demons challenge me,
but I tell them no.

During my first weeks at rehab,
the weekend boredom would be broken by bedside therapy.
When I still had a trach,
the therapist would come to my bedside
for 45 minutes
on either Saturday or Sunday.
But now, weaned from the trach,
I only get a miniscule 45 minute session
in the almost empty weekend gym.
45 minutes instead of the usual workweek's full day.
A paltry, short, insubstantial amount of time
against the wall of 48 hours.

Sunday mornings are the absolute worst.
I know I won't see anybody.
Everybody is at church.

Where is my church?

There is no Mass, no Eucharist,
no celebration of communal liturgy,
no magnificent choir,
no Word of the Lord or homily
to lift me up,
to reflect upon, to challenge me;
no love from my church community to validate,
support and strengthen me.

No church.

No Word.

Nothing but...aloneness.

One Sunday, we are promised an interfaith service.
I go, apprehensive but hungry,
only to find out that the host group has canceled out on us.
Again.

Left us flat.

But then, Monsignor shows up;
unexpected consolation in the midst of my desolation.
Feeling abandoned, rejected once more by the outside world,
I buzz off the elevator in my power chair,
and simultaneously,
Monsignor Liddy steps out of the neighboring elevator bank.

"What are you doing here on a Sunday morning?"
I query, incredulous,
not believing my eyes.

"I just came to see you," he replies in his gentle, always soothing voice.

"Well, let's go find a seat," I offer, and we settle into the day room.

I tell him how much I miss my youth ministry students
and how sad I feel knowing
that I won't be able to minister to them anymore.

"You're ministering every day from that chair," he replies.

I'm startled.
This was something I had never, ever considered.

But I knew he was right.

So many broken hearts had been opening up to me.
Wounded souls who had turned away from,
or who felt turned away by,
their churches.
Aunts who were mystified as to why
their God would allow
their twenty-something nephews
to become paraplegic.
And then there were those
who didn't verbalize any questions at all,
but if you looked hard enough,
their faces betrayed their souls' inner anguish.

We have been in pain together,
my fellow patients and I,
and in the midst of it
You were using me, Lord,
allowing me to lend a listening ear
or show compassionate concern
to a patient
or hurting family member.

You still use me, Lord.

As long as I pray and ask to be of service,
You let me partner with You…
somehow…
in quiet ways,
every day.

You've been restoring my soul.
I no longer live in the inner darkness
of my mood and spirit anymore,
as I did
when I was so sick and lost
in my first weeks here at rehab.
But even then,
unbeknownst to me at the time,
I was already being guided, nourished and nurtured
in the new life You granted me
as I learned to navigate
my new world
as a
quadriplegic, C4 - C7, incomplete.

Your love is all around.

You are there, Lord,
in the faces of pain and loss and sorrow,
and in the powerful healing connection
of a hug.

It is *Your* strength, Lord.

In You,
I can be that vessel of love,
that instrument of peace
that You've been calling me to be.
You spoke to me in my heart years before,
when I was at a very, very low point in my life.
In my arrogance and adherence to the gospel of self-sufficiency

I disparaged of ever being able to answer Your calling.
But Your words stayed in the shadows,
hidden in the deep recesses
of my soul.

My Lord,
for as long a time as I have left here on this earth,
let me be that vessel, that instrument,
so that others may know of
Your peace,
Your comfort,
Your compassion.
Help me reach them when they feel most alone,
as they struggle to make sense
of their situations
whether as a patient,
a parent,
a partner or loved one
undone by the overwhelming sense of loss,
of powerlessness,
of hurt.

Be there, Lord.
Help them find You.

Blaming and bitterness are no antidotes
for all the confusion, pain and suffering
in traumatically altered lives.
It is Your hope and Your connection
that are restorative.
They are grace,
embodied.

Amen.

Spirit's words to me

...Yes, I know, my earth is crying in its smug self-sufficiency, symptoms of thoughts that turn nowhere but in on themselves. And desperate souls, lost souls, hungry and poor souls. Humanity is seething with tears. I am so near child, yet many do not know. [Oh Lord, I am not worthy, I watered your presence down yesterday... eloquent I was not. Forgive me.] *Child, I already have. I am that God of compassion you wrote about before. Be my compassion. My spirit will give you the words, strength and power. Write, this is your summer of writing... I have so many more stories for you to tell my child many, many stories – some short images, poems. You will know. Just say yes to picking up your pen – and listening. I've called you home to me, tenderly. This is where your peace is my child, this is your peace... Enjoy the birds, seek out their song. Hear me in their symphonies, hear me...*

THE LEPER

*"The one who bears the sore of leprosy shall keep his garments rent
and his head bare...
He shall dwell apart, making his abode outside
of camp."* Leviticus 13:45-46

I only caught a glimpse of him that day, a mere glimpse. And in those seconds, I cringed, recoiling tightly inside myself.

I had to look away.

Everything about him was, well...just plain wrong!

He was standing there in his rags, looking so out of place, so lost and forlorn. Wispy, out-of-control, white hair seemed to sprout at odd angles all over his head. His skinny arms and spindly legs stuck out from under a pale blue hospital gown. Well, actually, it was two hospital gowns! The second was worn backwards in a poor attempt to make a modest bathrobe, except two long ties hung down from each side like worn-out, neglected strings.

I felt embarrassed, mortified, as if I had intruded into the bedroom of a barely dressed, strange man.

The dress codes in the gym were simple and made the therapists easy to spot. They all wore khakis, sneakers and brightly colored polo shirts embossed with our rehab's logo. The men's hair was always trim and neat, the women's hair was always shiny and, if long enough, in a ponytail. Each of our therapists were vibrant and healthy, walking about us with strength, grace and ease. They were bottomless wells of encouragement.

As for us patients, we were not the picture of health. The aides kept our hair neat if we couldn't manage it ourselves, but none of us looked like we had just come from the hair salon. Many of the fellows wore baseball caps and none looked as if they had recently seen a barber. Make-up belonged to another world; our faces were bare except for expressions of pain and struggle.

Male or female, we certainly didn't wear fitted khakis. Most of our families had been instructed to purchase sweatpants for us in a size larger than what we usually wore. This was not to hide figure flaws, but to make it easier for our aides to pull them over our brand new catheters and oversized pull-ups. All of us wore socks and sneakers, which the aides were well-versed in getting onto our paralyzed, unfeeling feet. And unless you were laboring with a therapist while learning to stand or to use a mobility device such as a walker, we were all using wheelchairs: standard, power, or sip-and-puffs.

And now, seemingly out of nowhere, there appears this scrawny man, standing among us in his flimsy cotton hospital gowns.

A patient, standing...without assistance! Where did this guy come from, anyway? Wait...was that guy even wearing shoes?

All I know is that he stood there in his half-dressed skinniness, sticking out like a sore thumb.

He wasn't one of us!

He really bothered me. Gave me the willies. He did not fit. He made me uncomfortable. I wanted him to go away. But since I couldn't make him go away, I turned away instead. Averting my eyes, I refused to look at him.

He was a misfit. A leper.

Later, I was ashamed. Why did I turn away? Frankly, I suspect this guy scared me at some level. But I still judged him harshly, without knowing him at all. That's when I realized that I saw him as nothing but a pauper, a leper, the ones you had to stay far away from *lest you catch what they had*.

Sorry, Jesus, I really fell down on that one, didn't I? And it was obvious: if you didn't look like me, then you became the "other," a threat to be ostracized, *lest I became like you*.

Lepers. Help me, Jesus.

Bless the lepers, Lord. I meet them everyday...and turn away. Instantly, sometimes subconsciously, instinctively, I judge. Every day, I feel threatened by those who don't look like me. Even as I sit in my wheelchair, with my deadened limbs and my useless, unfeeling fingers, how is it that I still manage to strive at being better than the "other"? For I, too, hunger to be loved and accepted. I, too, have been on the outside, "othered," long before my paralysis. I have been the too-tall and awkward kid on the playground in grammar school where kids talked behind my back and made fun of me. I have been told to sit in the "stupid row," when my brain was unable to process long division. I have been the kid in high school, excluded from the honors program where my friends were allowed to participate in amazing creative writing and painting classes and who were studying Shakespeare (something I was already reading on my own). I wanted to be 'better than,' overlooked and marginalized no more. But I was excluded by a learning disability long before such things were ever even heard of.

And Lord, I still remember the moment in that therapy gym when I heard my diagnosis stated, *'Tetraplegic C4-C7, Incomplete.'* You alone know how I felt when I heard that. I was devastated. *"Incomplete"...? You mean I can't even be a 'good enough' paralyzed person? That I'm STILL not good enough??*

More than anything, I want to be accepted and loved...just as I am.

Dear Lord....I AM the leper!

Teach me that Yours is the only love that is unwavering. Teach me that Yours is the only love that can sustain and strengthen me. Teach me that You accept and love me despite how others perceive or judge me.

Help me to understand that declaring myself as 'better than' the other, is just another cover up for the lie I keep telling myself, the one that tells me I am just not 'good enough.'

Love can heal the leper.

Your love can heal *me*, too.

Spirit's words to me

Jesus, what do you want?

To bring my comfort and compassion my child. Be my peace. It's not about preaching, it's about letting the weak hurt, bleed, some want to vomit their anger, but they will contain it. Call on my presence, my child...pray, my child, just pray. My presence and peace will be evident in you...keep your focus on me, keep your focus on me. Yes continue to write, my child, continue to write...

WAITING AND WRITING

By waiting and by calm you shall be saved,
In quiet and in trust your strength lies.
Isaiah 30:15

The waiting was dreadful.

Wait for someone to come and get you up.

Wait for someone to freshen you up, change you into daytime clothes.

Wait for them to get a Hoyer lift.

Wait to get you out of the bed, into the lift, into the chair.

Wait for them to push you out the door.

Wait in line for your meds.

Wait for them to push you to your assigned seat in the dining hall.

Wait for your tray of food to come.

Wait for someone to organize it on your plate, open the containers, cut your meat, open the great big bib, place it over your head and down your front.

Wait for breakfast to be finished.

Wait for someone to come and take you to the therapy gym.

By now, your body is beginning to internally scream with an eight out of ten pain scale due to an uncomfortable wheelchair.

And it's not even 10AM.

I lived in "wait."

Oh dear Lord, how I loathed it.

Ah, but Your sense of humor. It was Advent—the season of waiting, a time of soul preparation, a time to prepare our hearts for Your birth. I get it.

But I just couldn't take it anymore.

One evening, my dear friend had appeared almost magically at my bedside. I hadn't been expecting her visit. I knew that her time was almost always consumed by her Seton Hall administrative and academic duties; additionally, she was a greatly sought-after speaker for spiritual retreats. Although I thought I hadn't seen her since before my hospitalization, apparently, I was wrong. She gently told me that she had been visiting me since my admission to the ICU, way before my transfer to this nursing home. In her compassionate way, she redirected the discussion so as not to embarrass me or increase my confusion any further.

The usual 20 minute drive from campus had taken her almost 2 hours due to an accident and the resulting traffic jams; but still, she had come. Truly humbled by her efforts to see me, I felt such gratitude for her presence that night, a testament to her faithfulness and commitment to our friendship.

After a few minutes of light chatter, she eagerly presented me with an idea that I thought absolutely preposterous.

"Why don't you write a reflection for each day of Advent and by the end, you'll have 30 reflections – and a book!" Her face was filled with radiant light and her beautiful smile moved like a morning sun beam, aiming its love directly into my discouraged and hurting heart.

"A book?" I queried, *"A book?"*

"Sure," she said.

I thought she was nuts. Didn't she realize that my hands couldn't write? I could still only stab at the screen of my iPad, using a stylus attached to the stiff elastic cuff that my aides would slip over my hand. Mostly, I just read books from my Kindle app that the recreation therapist had so ingeniously installed. But, write a reflection a day? Now that was a skill set beyond my current ability.

But my dear friend just kept looking at me with that beatific smile, oblivious to any obstacles.

"Well, I'll think about it," I said, rather reluctantly. In spite of myself, I felt a small tingling of something. Something that didn't yet have a name. Maybe it was hope.

She didn't stay much longer after that.

"Can I do anything for you before I leave?" she asked.

I thought about it, then hesitated. I didn't want to bother her.

"Would you mind moving this little hair that seems to be laying across my right eye?"

"Why, of course." She did and we said our goodbyes.

Thoughts of my dear friend's visit, or more accurately, thoughts of her book idea, wandered through my mind as I lay there before falling asleep. "Waiting" was the first theme that came to mind, which is not surprising since that's what Advent is all about. Mary, pregnant and riding along the rocky road on a donkey's back, couldn't have felt much worse than the way I do sitting in that stupid wheelchair that doesn't fit. The theme stayed with me throughout the next day, but how was I going to come up with 29 more ideas for the rest of Advent? After two or three days of frustration, I gave up the waiting motif. I didn't think I would have anything else to say that would result in more than one paragraph, never mind 30 reflections. My dear friend did have a good idea, but she simply had too much faith in me!

In the prior month of November, my loyal friends from Seton Hall University - faculty, administrators and staff - had given me a "celebrate how far Maryann has come in her recovery" party. In a conference room at rehab, Mass was concelebrated with two of my priest friends and a pizza dinner with cake followed. The cake was a sight to behold! It featured my favorite Bible quote, "With God, all things are possible." (Matthew 19:26). In the center was a funny picture of Msgr Liddy on our Rome retreat. The picture was taken by someone looking up at the second floor retreat house window, where a smiling Msgr. Liddy was raising his hands in the famous greeting of the Pope to his people in the square below!

And then there were speeches and a presentation. One of the faculty presented me with a huge box that, after some good-natured heckling, they opened for me. From inside they pulled out a small box, a gift whose significance astounds me to this day. The faculty, administrator and staff community at Seton Hall had taken up a collection and graced me with... an iPad!

I'd seen my colleagues use them for photography while on the retreat in Rome the previous June. They must have remembered how I fell in love with the clarity and color the screens allowed. They must have remembered how much I loved taking pictures with my ever-present camera slung around my neck. Maybe they hoped I could shoot photographs with it one day and in the meantime, use it to at least read and perhaps learn to write or send them emails on my own!

I was overwhelmed with their generosity.

I was intrigued.

So, although I was the owner of a brand-new iPad, I didn't have a clue about what to do with it. The therapy team put their talents together and set me up with an elastic band that wrapped around my hand. They then inserted a stylus into the sleek leather holder in the palm side of the band and showed me how to maneuver around the internet. They installed a Kindle for reading and a voice activated system into which I could dictate.

Wait...dictate? Ahh! A new way to write! That gift from my friends who believed in me became my bridge back, or perhaps the gateway, to a new future.

And now here I was in the nursing home, a month or so later and my dear friend was suggesting that I write daily reflections. Although it had been an idea born out of her benevolence, initially I didn't think it could happen. Yet somehow, the idea planted itself deep within my soul, took root and began to grow.

By now, my iPad was my constant companion. Once my aides had gotten me settled into my chair, they would place my iPad upon my lap and slip the adaptive cuff around my hand, slide the stylus into the palm slot and carefully wrap my stiff and tightly curled fingers around it. For the rest of my free time during the day, I could effectively poke and stab away on my iPad screen for as long as my arm would allow. Or at least until the next scheduled activity required the dismantling of the carefully constructed contraption!

This piece of technology continued to open more and more worlds to me. Since my admission to the nursing home, I had learned to play Mandisa's "Good Morning" song every morning after I was wheeled into the line to wait for my meds. It was a fun way to pep people up! Also, I had not been able to attend weekly Mass since my hospitalization started five long months before. This iPad had allowed me to discover the Sunday scripture readings so that, at least, I could read them on my own. And now I was given another inspiration! If I could make the iPad understand what I was saying, then maybe I *could* write some kind of reflection. So I asked my speech therapist if she could work with me on my dictation app. She was delighted to comply.

Pretty soon, I had a purpose.

I'm writing a book, I thought to myself. Soon enough, I began to say it out loud.

"I'm writing a book!"

You know me, Lord. You knew I needed a purpose. You knew how I've always wanted to write a book, yet, You also knew that I felt I had nothing significant enough in my life to write about.

But now I did. I'd tell my story!

And write, I did. Every day in the nursing home I'd try to write something. I continued to write on a daily basis when I was finally able to return to rehab in January. Most of the time, my dictation came out so garbled that I couldn't understand what I'd written. Still, I persisted. From all that incomprehensible dictation, I advanced to being able to write on my iPad. With the help of my stylus strapped to my hand, I tapped on my iPad keyboard, one laborious letter at a time.

So, yes, I was a bit off of the track of my dear friend's original, spiritually targeted suggestion, however, I was filled with a new sense of purpose. *I'd write MY story so I could help other people going through their challenges.*

The idea empowered me, gave me something I had lost and completely forgotten about. Maybe it was a sense of direction or strength, a gentle nudge that gave me that feeling I had forgotten about. That feeling, so long elusive, the inklings of which first began to stir when my dear friend mentioned her book idea to me—I had a sense of it now. It went by the name of...*hope.* All of my former identities seemed to have been steamrolled flat to nothing on the newly paved road that was now my life, but yet, I had found hope. My experiences could help somebody else! I felt like I was somebody again.

After my discharge from rehab to home, I had a rocky month of adjustment. But the writing goal was still there. Soon enough, I started outpatient therapy on Tuesdays and Thursdays, so on the alternating weekdays, I made it my business to write. My home aide would drive me up my street and across the busy county road to the Seton Hall campus. Once there, she would help transfer me from the car to the chair, so that I could "wheel" across campus. To the uninitiated, my way of "wheeling" must have looked pretty odd. Although it was a standard wheelchair, my arms did not have the strength, nor my hands the grip, to wheel it. Instead,

I would move forward by alternately hitting the heels of my feet down, one after the other.

My first destination was always noon Mass in the chapel and, filled with determination, I would make my long way across campus. Once I arrived at the chapel, my initial challenge would be to get myself up the ramp. In the beginning, I needed to wait for some help to make it up the steep incline. But eventually, I was able to do it on my own. With all the power I could muster, I would use my weak arm to grab onto the railing and *pull* with all my might. Ahh, that would get me forward by at least 3 inches! In due course, all of those inches would pay off and get me up the ramp, where the next formidable obstacle awaited me: the door. In the summer, one of the outside doors would usually be open, but inside the vestibule, the tightly sealed inner doors would keep the air conditioning in....and people without arm strength, out. And so, I would sit and wait till someone came along that could help me. After Mass it would be the same thing; I would have to wait for someone to open the heavy doors for me. Then down the ramp I would go and on to my final destination: the library.

The library had been a sanctuary for me since I was a little girl and it was no different now. I would find an accessible desk and proceed to write on my iPad for the rest of the afternoon, poking away with my stylus attached to my hand cuff.

And write, I did.

Two years later, just before Easter, I finished my second rewrite. A great sense of self-satisfaction washed over me; I felt certain that my book was done.

But then, Lord, in Your not very subtle way, You changed everything. In my morning prayer, You told me: *Readers will find comfort as I renew My presence through your story of hope and connection, passion and suffering.*

It was time to put the focus back on You—to let You lead and design the book. The story of Your comfort had been pushed way into the background. Instead, it had become a story of *my* hardships and triumphs, putting *me* in the spotlight. It was all about *me* first, oh and, of course, about how "I" could help someone else facing adversity as well. You, my sweet Lord, had become an afterthought.

In other words, my "memoir" had to go.

So, back to my dear friend's words on that one winter night in Advent long ago. Your message to write from the angle of spirituality was there. I had just missed the point!

Lord, lead my writing now, so Your lost and suffering ones may learn to see glimpses of grace all around them.

And in Your words, *"Indeed, brokenness may be the human condition; healing is the divine."*

Let the healing begin.

Spirit's words to me

My child, let my peace reign in your heart, fill you with my compassion and my grace. My child, remain open to me. Tell me your desires, aches and needs – I am always, always here for you. I am glad that you want to make more room for me, for my words and stories... Ahh, my sweet, dear child, my mission to you is clear - to bring my comfort to suffering souls - and my way is clear as well – write and be present to me. You will know peace, you will know fulfillment and enjoy. You will see souls shine... sometimes their light is so hidden under pain and anger. My words will heal them child, my mercy and compassion. They will only know pain and darkness - fruitless – cut off from me. Remain in me, remain open. Write like you've never written before. Write, write, write.

SURRENDER

"When I called, you answered me;
You build up strength within me."
Psalm 138:3

Waiting was dreadful.

I was trapped in a mesh of misery since my first day at the nursing home, a mesh that was threatening to strangle the light and life out of my spirit.

I was scared, frightened, miserable and alone.

Or, so I thought.

What was I doing in a nursing home? I didn't fall and break my hip at 80, nor get senile overnight. Six months ago, I had become a quadriplegic, C4 - C7, paralyzed from the neck down, requiring full assistance for personal care and rehabilitation. Due to insurmountable insurance obstacles, I was taken out of my highly specialized care center and re-assigned to an in-house care facility to await the turn of the calendar year. So, here I was, feeling abandoned and increasingly terrified, surrounded by a bunch of lonely old people.

The hours in this place grew intolerably long as I languished through the unending hours of the night in my bed or crumpled in the discomfort of my uncomfortable wheelchair. With growing despondency, I felt misery contaminating me, seeping into my bones. I knew I was dying here.

Maryann was wasting away.

Did I pray fervently to God for peace and patience and strength? No. I was terrified and couldn't believe that God would put me here. Surely, this must be some kind of cruel, sick joke. I felt totally separated from God. I could feel none of His grace. I could feel none of His compassion. I only felt as if I had been left for dead.

Oh, how I ached for the days in the rehab gym with therapists who pushed, prodded, challenged and celebrated. They had called me a rock star.

But here, I felt like a nobody.

As a result of my injury, I had already lost my former self, my physical freedom, my roles and identity; but now I was losing everything I had been working so hard at my rehab to build up again. I was devastated. Soon I began to burn with an anger and a confusion that I was too scared to even acknowledge. Terror consumed my being. I grew increasingly convinced that I had been abandoned, my newly found voice, once silenced by a ventilator, was now completely ineffective and unheard, my paralyzed body unprotected.

I had arrived at this nursing home on the eve of the first Sunday of Advent, the beginning of the liturgical season that marks the four weeks leading to Christmas. In the past, it was a time I had used to reflect, to find the places where I might go deeper and discover what God wanted to do inside my heart.

But, not now. I felt awful. Instead of quiet reflection, I was immersed in dread. There was no anticipation of a sacred birth, or of sacred and secular preparation for a wonderful and renewing feast day. Already, a few miserable, gut-wrenching weeks had passed and now my soul was in agony, tortured, overcome with an abject terror that deadened my once-joyful spirit. I felt abandoned and alone, in a paralyzed body from which I had no escape. I could not go on like this anymore.

I had hit rock, solid, bottom. I was *done*.

And then, one night, in that deep darkness that had devoured my soul, a prayer suddenly broke through, released out of that cloying abyss. It was from a paragraph I had memorized many years before, somehow making its way out of the depths of my disquiet and desperation. I began to recite what I could remember of it, slowly and painstakingly at first and then, carefully, thoughtfully.

"Nothing, absolutely nothing, happens in God's world by mistake. Unless I accept life completely on life's terms, I cannot be happy."

I let that sink in for a few minutes.

Then, without warning, I was forced to confront a devastating paradigm-shifting, identity-stripping thought.

Maybe I'll never walk again.

Hearing those words come from deep within my being was, to say the least, shocking. Admitting it to be truth was nothing short of terrifying. It meant letting go of the strongest hope in my heart. It meant that I had to give up every last shred of my identity, every last shard of my plans and my hopes, to my Creator.

Ok Lord, I thought. *Is this what You want? If You want me to be here for now, then ok. Whatever You want…*

To say the beginning of this surrender was difficult would be an understatement. More accurately, every step consumed my very being. Everything was being taken away from me. My dreams, my hopes…they were all I had. And there were many:

I was *going to* walk again.

I was *going to* run again.

I was *going to* build houses with my youth ministry kids and young adults again.

I was *going to* run retreats.

I was *going to* walk up to campus from my home and greet my favorite security guard at the gate.

I was *going to* walk across the campus green.

I was *going to* walk into the chapel.

I was *going to* learn to walk just as my grandbaby soon would.

I was *going to* carry her, cuddle her, push her in a stroller and chase after her.

But now…?

I…was going to?

Maybe, just maybe, *I wasn't.* Maybe *I was not* going to walk, run, or carry my grandbaby. Maybe *I* was *not* going to do any of those things *I* had dreamed about.

On the heels of that revelation followed another heart-convicting realization…one that rebuked me to my core. These had all been my plans, the grand scheme, the meta-narrative of my new life.

And then it came. The great reckoning: MY way was not working.

Lord, I guess I thought *I* was running Your show. I had been trying to steal Your role. It had become embarrassingly clear that I thought *"I"* was the director of Your universe.

Sigh.

Finally, I began to consider defeat. Reluctantly, I let go of my dreams and ambitions from rehab. My pride and false sense of self-sufficiency were completely — and utterly — stripped away.

OK, Lord, I'm here. I give up, I'm all Yours.

And I was.

Over the next few nights and days, the heavy cloak of pessimism and negativity which had enrobed my being began to ease its way off of my shoulders. My dismal demeanor began its slow transformation. My heart started to open, slowly, slowly, ever so cautiously.

Before I surrendered to God, I had been centered and focused only upon myself. I had completely lost sight of any opportunity, however big or small, to be of service. No wonder I had been so miserable: I had been making my life all about me!

Lord, through my surrender, You graced me with the brand new lenses I would now use to see my life. I never knew my vision could become so weak and blurred. Until now, I could not even recognize that I hadn't been able to see Your real purpose or Your presence anywhere.

But now, with my brand new lenses, I could.

Until this moment, I hadn't realized I was afraid of being forgotten by the outside world, all of my past achievements discarded like dust in the wind. It was this fear, burrowing itself deep inside of me, that had created a strong divide between me and my fellow nursing home residents. Ever so slowly, I started to reach out. Now that my eyes were opening, I found myself falling in love with all of these quiet, eccentric old people.

Our primary gathering place was in the therapy gym and without much forethought, I found myself beginning conversations with my fellow sojourners. Light and only touching the surface at first, our dialogue began to go deeper as we grew more comfortable with each other; my heart, initially frozen shut in fear, began to open to the light of love. I know now that it was Your Spirit, Lord, urging me through my intuition, leading me to begin to reach out. Through these quick interactions, I started to discover the astonishing strength and beauty in these new friends of mine. Especially in the women.

One place where You led me to reach out was at the table of women with whom I shared all of our meals. I had noticed that there were a few Catholic women among us and I began to wonder if they missed attending

Mass and hearing the scriptures read as much as I did. One day, while I was relentlessly poking away with the stylus on my iPad, I discovered how to access the Sunday Mass readings. Suddenly I thought: *would the other Catholic women be willing to gather together with me on Sunday to read the Scriptures together?*

Finally, I managed to pull up my courage and ask the women if we could meet in one of their rooms to read the Sunday scripture. Although hesitant at first, with a bit of friendly persuasion, they agreed. We met in the largest of our rooms, easiest for our three wheelchairs. Once we were settled, I pulled up the Sunday scriptures from the iPad on my lap and read them aloud. Hearing Your words was so comforting to me Lord.

I know in their quiet ways, Lord, they were thankful to hear the Word...and so was I. Somehow, our hearts were lighter. I didn't realize how much I had missed them—and all the life lessons and the sense of security I used to receive from listening to them. For at least a few moments, we were being fed by a power greater than ourselves. We were being fed by our God whom we recognized in the scriptures and by a Mother God so yearning to bend down and feed the hungry souls of her children crying out in their nest.

And as you fed my hungry soul Lord, I could feel my surrendered heart begin to slowly open. As I gave in to Your love, my whole being was beginning to soften. Instead of being consumed with discontent, there was a new space inside of me that was receptive, waiting, suddenly ready to reach out to those around me in love.

Yes, I was still paralyzed and no longer in my beloved and familiar rehab hospital. Yet, I was also getting to know You and trust You in a very different way. I was finding You as I forgot about me and began to love those around me.

You opened my heart and gave me a new vision, a new hope...a new life.

I felt alive again. It was the act of my surrender to You—my surrender to Your deep, abiding grace—that gave me new life. That's all that it took: discovering once again that *my* ways don't work. I needed to concede my willfulness to the power who created me out of love, who is love...and who is in love with me.

Take care of me, Lord. Change my fearful and limited vision.

Spirit's words to me

My child, indeed I have been revealing much to you. As you learn to listen to me, you will become — as you are becoming — more aware of the heart of the matter. I have promised you a new vision... My child, you are whole in me. Trust in me and my healing presence. You are a fine writer — it is a gift I have given you. You are a fine chaplain as well. Indeed, all is well. Ask for more clarity and I will give it to you my child. Yes...there are so many more stories - leave me the space to tell them to you.

THE AGONY IN THE GARDEN...
AND OTHER PLACES

"Then going out he went, as was his custom,
to the Mount of Olives...
"Father, if you are willing, take this cup away from me;
Still, not my will but yours be done."
And to strengthen him
an angel from heaven appeared to him.
He was in such agony and he prayed so fervently
that his sweat became like drops of blood
falling on the ground."
Luke 22:39-44

Lord, I never asked You to take my cup from me.

Although I was bereft of energy and direction in the beginning, it was Your grace and the power of prayer that gave me strength beyond my own. All I knew to do was what I was taught to do, which was to say *"Thy will – not mine – be done."*

Your grace spared me from asking that simple and profound question which continues to haunt so many patients and their families in the night: *why me?*

I never asked.

"And to strengthen him, an angel from heaven appeared to him." (Lk. 22:43)

You sent me so many angels when I was at rehab.

They came to me deep in the night when I needed help the most, arriving at my bedside in soft-soled shoes and scrubs. Quiet, gentle aides. Somewhere in the beginning, my elimination raged out of control because heavy-duty meds were being pumped into my worn-out body to fight the pneumonia that had invaded it.

Different aides would come to clean me up, sometimes three or four times a night. They cleaned me, changed me, changed my bed, my linens, all with only soothing and kind words. One slight disparaging word, one hint of a complaint could have added to my shame and destroyed any threads of dignity I had left. Instead, their patient, kind ways afforded me dignity, afforded me grace.

Angels.

Night after night, more gentle angels would come to my bedside to give me my meds. Softly and tenderly, these nurses would call my name as I slept. They did not want to frighten me. Hungry for home, for academia, for the familiarity of Seton Hall and my friends on the nursing faculty, I grilled and interrogated each of these poor souls between my med doses. They were always patient with me as I asked time and time again, "And did you get your nursing degree at Seton Hall?"

Kindness....Your angels were always kind.

And they accepted my kindness, too.

My rehab hospital wasn't the only place with night angels. Each night at the nursing home, I waited for my angel aide, praying for endurance when I was in so much pain. She would start working with her assigned patients at 11 pm, finally getting to my room around 12:30 or 1:00 AM. She was the person most adept at positioning and turning my paralyzed body. Although she always brought another aide to help, it was unnecessary. Nothing could replace the experience and training she had gained years before, working with spinal cord injury patients at another facility.

My nurses in the night here at the nursing home were beings of great kindness, too. I looked forward to the times they would care for me. Without them, I don't know how far I would have spiraled downward, since I was being swallowed by so much of my own misery, so much fear and loss. Through their professionalism, their perspective and their kindness indeed, Lord, You sent them to strengthen me.

Their love was essential to my healing.

Your angels continued to appear in the evenings and nights on the last leg of my journey when I returned to the rehab hospital. They changed me, got me into bed, adjusted me and the pillows, turned me, ministered to my sin-sick soul.

One Tuesday morning a few years after I was back home again, You showed me something while I was praying the Sorrowful Mysteries. I realized that an angel came to You, but did not take Your pain away – You prayed more fervently and sweated harder! The angel didn't say *Sure, gotcha, only kidding, there's been a change of plans, you don't have to go through with this, no dying tomorrow.*

No paralysis tomorrow.

No bowel program or catheter to contend with tomorrow.

"His sweat became like drops of blood falling to the ground" ...and that was *after* You had given up Your will, after the angel came to strengthen You.

My episodes of pain at night could be blinding. They would both blind-side me, coming seemingly out of nowhere and physically blind me with their intensity. Usually, I would try to keep praying and singing through the pain. But then, my angels of the night would come. Some people describe Your presence as a certain sense or impression. But for me, Your presence was always in the real physical presence of a nurse or aide. Sometimes You reached me through the compassion in the voice of a nurse who would have to tell me my meds weren't due for another hour. When my leaden body was left unmoved or in an incorrect position for just a little too long, leaving me consumed by the fires of agony from the rawness of my misfiring nerves, You would send someone to reposition my torso and limbs in just the right way and release me from my torture.

Indeed, I learned that the pain would pass.

But not Your angels.

They were always there.

Spirit's words to me

Write a story of your pain much deeper child – disappointment, disillusionment, doubt - that is where your heart is – my readers will understand then – like Thomas as a prototype for the doubter, your situation is not unique among families that have been fractured by serious illness and certainly by alcoholism. Write for me child, that my comfort may reach the lost and stumbling souls, at their wits end. Oh, dear Lord I want to help those other mothers - and it seems so unfair that they can't find you right there in the hospital – *Teach them to see me my child. You bring me to them in the midst of their pain – you will bring me in the Eucharist, in your presence – which is my presence – and in your books which will be picked up in odd hours or handed to someone somewhere who is hurting. That is why it is imperative that you show your pain, or identify it in others. No more 'news reporting' my child, the heart of the matter, the holes in my hands and my side helped Thomas, the stories I will give you and remind you of will teach some hurting soul in a hospital room or at home feeling so aggrieved, alone, overwhelmed, terrified and sad. My dear child, it is not for you to see the big picture – just stay in the now with me, in my ever-present healing grace.*

MORNING GLORIES/MOMENTS

It was time to start a new day.

By the last month of my hospitalization, nights were still continuing to prove difficult and long. In what had become my nighttime ritual for the past four months, I laid on my bed looking up at the big clock on the wall, the second hand literally crawling its way around the circle. Click after click, each minute was excruciatingly painful in its slowness. Being turned every two hours was the only relief I had from the endless hours alone and unable to sleep or move. I felt so trapped in my body, in that bed, feeling as if the night would never, *ever* come to an end. I did not know that I was in a constant state of hypervigilance, from my then as yet undiagnosed ICU-associated PTSD.

But when my daytime aide finally came in to greet me in the morning, I knew I had survived another night. The day's invitation to live in the new light was beckoning.

I was ready. And the good Lord provided.

The Great Spirit, the Artist and Creator of the universe, saw fit to feed my soul with glimpses of what I so dearly missed: nature at its winter's best. One of these gifts was the morning of the pink trees.

I thought I was seeing things.

My final hospital room was on the south wing at rehab. The beautiful windows in my room may have been sealed shut against the cold winter air, but they gave me a clear view of something the Lord knew I hungered for: *trees*.

Perhaps there were only a few, but in my mind's eye, they were a forest. Since we were now in early February, all of the leafless trees were dormant and still, resting in their winter's slumber. Without an evergreen in sight, they formed a solid wall of gray and brown, often against a barely visible blue sky.

On this particular morning, I awoke to quite a surprise. As my eyes slowly opened and I glanced at my beloved trees, I saw something that seemed surreal. I could only stare, mesmerized by the vision outside my windows. As far as my eyes could see, every one of the trees was blushing pink.

I had to ask myself: *Were my meds causing my colorful vision?* But then I realized that no, the trees were really and truly pink. For a few barely discernible moments, God's grandeur of the new morning soothed my soul. It was the Artist God's sunlight, streaming, filtered across the top of rehab hospital's rooftops, that had turned those trees pink.

A silent dance of color, transformative color, giving life in the deadness of winter. The perfect watercolor vision took my breath away.

A sacred gift, Lord. Only You were capable of that.

These were the moments that satiated my soul. I knew they would have to suffice for now. I didn't think I'd be cross-country skiing or snowshoeing in my beloved Adirondacks anytime soon.

But then, there were the mornings that weren't so idyllic. My latest roommate always kept the television on. Her favorite morning station devoted itself to pummeling the current presidential administration, stopping at nothing to sensationalize or moralize. So, after the morning routine of being tidied up, dressed and put into my power chair, I ate my breakfast. Then, I made haste to leave my room.

I needed to escape the relentless nastiness and noise.

Fortunately, in addition to the beautiful windows and view in my room, I had the pleasure of being at the end of the hall. As soon as I buzzed my power chair out of my room, a bank of windows, floor to ceiling, awaited me. Their view granted me access to more food for my soul: an early morning view of trees and sunshine.

Here, I found a place of refuge from the TV's incessant noise. After a few mornings gazing out at God's grandeur, my quiet spot transformed into a place for prayer. I wasn't yet savvy enough to use meditation or reflection apps on my iPad and a prayer book with pages to turn was still beyond my ability level. But God knew and heard my heart.

So in this new place of quiet, I gave thanks for all of my caregivers. I gave thanks for the entire rehab hospital team. I gave thanks for all of those people who prayed for me. I was able to pray for all of my fellow spinal cord injury patients and other residents on our floor. For these, especially, who were hurting from all of their sudden losses and challenges and so much in need of prayer. For all of them, I prayed.

During one of these mornings, Mother Nature provided a breathtaking ice show. I could see long, lovely rows of trees, perhaps twenty or thirty of them. Every single skinny, young tree had every single skinny bare limb covered with ice. Frozen crystals gleamed in the sun, twinkling and flashing their diamond white lights in a breathtaking display of beauty.

I sat in a new kind of deep down stillness, completely entranced.

A thousand lights, a thousand twinkling lights, gleaming in the morning's majestic sunrise.

Dear Lord, You were feeding my starving soul, in small doses. You knew my undernourished soul was hungry for nature's blissful bounty of fresh air, wind, snow, sunshine and rain. You knew how much I missed running, deep in the silent woods on dark, slippery, muddy trails.

You fed me.

Thank you for Your kindness, Lord. Thank you, Great Spirit, Artist and Creator of the universe. Thank you for taking such special care of me.

With all my being...*thank You.*

Spirit's words to me

...Listen deeply to my spirit, indeed it is time for you to let go of your plans, for I have more for you to do – my ways will reach more people in a better way than you can see. Yes, give me your chaplaincy, your education, your writing, give it all to me and say yes, that your heart may hear the whole of it.

Your book is larger than what you thought, give it to me, give your whole heart to me, all your hidden thoughts and desires for I have created you, my little one, my precious one. Let me speak to you and through you – write, study, teach, reach, sit still with me, sit still with hurting families, sit still. There is so much more – let me handle the details.

Stay open, let me feed you in your nest. Come rest and curl up with me. Let me feed you, nurture you, nourish you and teach you. You are my precious one. Do not be afraid.

SINGING

"Fear is useless - what is needed is trust."
Luke 8:50

I had to do a lot of trusting.
I trusted in You, Lord
and all the ones You sent
to take care of me.
I quickly learned to read the moods of my aides;
I didn't want anybody to be rough with me.
Not that they would ever be,
It was just my terrible fear.
I was completely and utterly helpless—
and yes, I was probably completely terrified.
I had to trust in You.

The singing helped.
It added levity.
It was sheerly for survival
through the pain when I was turned in the nights.
It was also in the core of my being
that I had to be the nice "Hobbie girl"
(there were five siblings, four girls, one boy)
I was raised to be.
I couldn't disappoint my late parents
and the good Sisters who educated me.
They raised me in charity.
They raised me to be kind.
I did not want to hurt anyone with my words or behavior.

Singing is one of my earliest memories
when I "came to" at rehab.
Singing was not my own idea;
it couldn't have been.
Who in their right mind would sing
when they were out of their mind with pain?
You knew that I just couldn't bear to be
yet another patient
who yelled or cursed at the poor aides
when they had to move our heavy, hurting bodies.
Our pain - *my* pain -
was not their fault.

I refused to yell.
I made a solemn pledge
to sing through all of the searing, burning pain
that was instantaneous
whenever and wherever I was touched.

And, sing, I did.

But not with the ease or gusto I used to have.
First off, my strong choir voice was gone.
I barely had the voice—or the breath—
for any sustained talk at all.
And then there was my repertoire.
Before I got hurt,
my repertoire consisted of an expansive
lifelong assemblage of church songs,
musicals, camp songs, folk songs and lullabies.
There had to have been hundreds of songs in my brain.

But, now, as I was being moved
every two hours throughout the night
every raw nerve screamed in protest
at every single touch.

I could *not* scream,
I *would not* scream
so...I sang.
But due to the level of pain,
my brain's vast storage system of music
went into shutdown...
I could only recall a few songs.
I didn't have the strength or the wherewithal to think
beyond them.

So here was the musical program:
First, there were the two opening lines from *Oklahoma's*
"Oh, What A Beautiful Mornin".
And then, two lines of a hymn that no one,
including our church music director/friend,
had ever heard of
(and he has been a church musician since he was 11 years old).
Finally, there was
a battered version of one of his arrangements
of a "Gloria" from Sunday mass.

That was it.
No more and no less.
And when the pain was sustained,
the repertoire in my mind just repeated itself.

In fact, one night-nurse
admitted that she had sung
the "Gloria"
all the way home.
She knew it well
because for three nights she had to perform
a very painful procedure on me.
On the third night she said to me,
"I have to confess,
if that was me laying in that bed

having this procedure done,
you would've heard me yelling
all the way down the hall!"

Oh my sweet Lord...
It was Your grace.
Nothing but grace.
It was You that gifted me with song
through all that pain.

And all of those prayers, Lord...
I know
it was the strength of all of those prayers
from my family,
my church,
and the Seton Hall University community
that sustained me.

Bless those aides, Lord;
don't let them down.
Remind them that their work can be Your presence
for the lonely, sick and afraid.

Help them to be respected,
to respect themselves,
to be paid well and to be listened to.
For they are the backbone
of every hospital.

Thank you for the music.
Thank you for the grace.
Thank you for Your never-ending,
always present
love.

So be it.
Amen.

Spirit's words to me

Just stay close to me, my child. Indeed, I know the desires of your heart — I put them there! Celebrate your success, your biggest success, heart open to see my presence. Oh my child, so many of my children are lost, trapped in their misery, feeling like victims, powerless victims without me. They need to see differently. Yes, your eyes got infected — you were not seeing as I wanted you to see. Look to me, the healer, the creator of owls, salamanders and butterflies, hummingbirds, woodpeckers — my animals all around the globe. Yes, my child, I want you to be able to drink in their beauty. Do not hold back nor go off course now. I am right here for you. Focus on me, call on my presence to sustain you. That is why you can succeed and go forth, I have transformed you, given you a new awakening of your heart, so that you could see beyond your body's limits. Without those limits, you have lost me. We are home together. Write, ride, dream, yes indeed, you will have your mountains, sky and trees, streams — so you can fill your soul with my beauty — and reach others who are so desperately in need. Your daughter belongs to me. Let go even more deeply that I may heal both your souls. You are not the same person, child. Let her be with me. Read your book, ask your questions — and let go and write, write, write.

THE MOTHER

She hovers at the bedside, or outside the doors of the therapy gym. She uses whatever free moments she can find to check in with her family waiting at home or to relentlessly negotiate with the insurance company. If you ask her what day of the week it is, she probably wouldn't know.

She's been living in timeless suspension since the day of the accident, not that she can tell you the time, place or circumstance.

But that was the day her life changed forever. Her young adult, just graduated or off at college, or newly graduated and off at work, suffered an injury that reduced her to a new kind of dependency not known since infancy.

And this mother will not leave her child's side for anything.

She's followed her child through the treacherous waters of the ICU. Her child survived; and now, in the rehabilitation hospital, the mother is there cheering for them, staying in the background so that her child can learn new forms of independence. She weeps for them, her heart breaking for what was, what now is and what will be along the way and for the pain that she witnesses. She only allows the luxury of tears when she can silently weep to herself in the night, on the cot next to her young adult's hospital bed, or when she can find the rare private hiding spot.

She advocates and, always, she prays for them.

This mother is wounded, deeply. She feels so powerless, so lost and alone. Her spouse, (if she has one), is back at work. Neighbors are pitching in to help on the home front, relatives and friends show up when they can, which is most often only on the weekends.

But even the visiting friends can be a challenge, too. They don't know what to say, deeply uncomfortable and visibly distressed at the sight of their friend mutilated, a ghost of their former self. Mom watches and senses their shock, tries to encourage her son, her daughter, who is now more than keen in the art of reading those startled faces with their *"I'm out of here"* expressions underscoring their already awkward and strained chatter. Despite her repeated invitations, subtle hints and outright appeals, she watches, powerless, as the visitors decline first in number, then in frequency and her heart breaks even more. These bewildered friends scurry back to their familiar worlds of study and work, leaving the unbearably strange new life of their old friend behind. Mom has to struggle to find new footing. She stretches her core emotions to understand, to accept that youths have to move on. She's angry, but the anger merely masks her own fear...*what will become of her child?*

And somehow, as she learns to carefully tread over the shattered glass and broken shards of this new territory, she comes to understand, at some level, that this will work out. That the old definitions of identity, sports, school, work, won't fit anymore.

She remembers when her child was a little one, growing out of their sweet little shoes, mastering language, friendships, relationships, gradually emerging into their strong, confident twenty, thirty-something-year-old self. And then she thinks about what this young adult has just survived, how they were brought to the brink of death and then...they came back again.

She wants to believe that there *will* be a new life for her child. The constant encouragement of their health care team, doctors, nurses and nurses' aides and every imaginable therapist, begins to sink in deep down somewhere and strengthen her, too. Mom is learning a new language, a language that speaks Hope. A language that listens beyond the surface words, that recognizes their son's, their daughter's grit and uplifts the soul shining through.

And so, Mom camps out at her child's bedside. At night, she monitors every breath and moan and blood pressure, goes to sleep on the cot saying her prayers. She helps when she is allowed, taking on some of her child's personal care, asking questions, wanting to, needing to, learn. She queries the doctors, pesters for answers and looks to the nurses as her lifeline.

She is living in limbo...that in-between state, where the tiniest flicker of hope hovers, not quite ready to land. But then a sudden wind blows through, unbidden, threatening to extinguish that tiny spark: the challenge of an infection, insurmountable insurance issues, home health care or home accessibility issues, problems simmering then erupting in the neglected "others"—children, spouse—who are feeling forgotten and left out at home. With any of these, that meager, already flickering light of hope can weaken, falter and fade just a little more.

And always...always there are the questions that persist, the ones that relentlessly rob her of her sleep at night, demanding answers she's not even sure she wants to know. *How much recovery can they expect? What will it look like? Can her child go back to college, job, or return to the brand-new career now so rudely interrupted?*

She learns to think differently, in the tiniest of increments, measuring progress not by where her child was before the accident, but by the progress they've made since their admission to rehab. One little eye movement, the tiniest finger twitch, a swallow, a breath on their own... she celebrates.

But Mom needs to be celebrated, too, Lord. She's worn out, weary from the battles.

Sometimes she feels so alone.

Mercy, Lord. This shocked and wounded caregiver needs Your mercy.

If only the Moms could connect with each other. To whisper their fears and their trials to each other, to share their grief, their hopes, frustrations and desires. There is hope in that connection. I've seen it. I've seen hope born when a Mom has shared her worries and doubts with other Moms and with patients in the weekly spirituality group. They know they're understood.

I have witnessed hope where I was able to give communion in their child's room week after week...the broken body of Christ reaching out to the broken ones.

This is Your mercy, Lord. *This is Your mercy.*

I've seen hope in the mothers who know they can trust me. They know me from bringing them the Eucharist every week in their child's room, or have gotten to know me as I waited for my own therapy in the outpatient waiting room. They open their hearts to me in a stolen hallway moment, pain lining the deep creases on their face. They discover empowerment in knowing that they are heard and understood, in the hugs and the tears of release. That connection, that feeling of being understood, is a very, very powerful balm for the soul. That connection is healing, Lord and it builds the resilience their wounded spirits so need...

This connection, this resilience, Lord. This *is* Your mercy.

You are the catalyst for the connection, Lord. Yours is the power behind the hope...hope born of loss, of the death of what was, the uncertainty, the crush of what is now. And You are the grace that gives birth to the new and different life that has yet to reveal itself.

Some of those Moms depend on You, God! They storm the heavens for Your protection and grace. Some are beyond angry at You, but they'll accept the love around them.

They don't have to know that it comes from You.

You *are* their mercy, Lord...You ARE mercy!

And You are love.

Bless them, Lord.

Protect them. Their journeys are so difficult.

Help the Moms, Lord. Help Your Moms tend Your broken, grown children entrusted to their care once again.

They can't do it alone.

They need Your mercy, Lord. They need...*You.*

Feed My sheep? Yes, Lord. Just show me how.

Spirit's words to me

My child, I saved you for my Word and my presence. Do not hesitate to serve me or speak for me. My words are in your heart; indeed, I am making room for the new. Look to me for guidance. Your writing has entered a new phase. Be open...Pray for peace for all the people I have placed in your heart. Oh my child, I grieve for you and my lost ones, I want you all back in my love, in my light, in my embrace. Let me remake you, that you may stand strong and steadfast and do my will. Go on now child, go and prepare for mass and the new truths I will uncover for you. Ask me for my words, I will give them to you. Fear not, my little one, you are safe in me.

THE SHOELACE

The campus was deserted.

It was a Friday afternoon in the middle of summer. My husband had dropped me and my trusty wheelchair off at our customary spot by the flagpoles, at the foot of the handicapped ramp by the campus' front entrance. After he opened my wheelchair and we bade each other goodbye, I positioned myself behind the chair. I gripped the handles as best as my hands would allow and began my slow crawl up the access ramp. I knew that my husband would not drive away until he saw that I was safe and sound on level ground. I grinned, knowing that he was waiting behind me, loyal and patient to the end. Pausing when I reached the top, I let out a deep sigh as I heard him drive away and turned my attention to my walk. The wheelchair was my source of stability as I gained strength and my transportation when I needed to sit again.

As my cautious and uneasy gait began to fall into a slow but measured rhythm, I began to relax a little bit. My eyes could not get enough of the lush green that surrounded me. With every breath, I drank in the calm, the color. Trees in their fullness, beds of brightly-colored flowers everywhere, a paradise for the heart, for the nature lover like me who had spent the last three seasons sealed inside soul-numbing institutions. For many years and for many seasons, I had watched the grounds crew take tender, loving care of every inch of the lawns, pulling weeds by hand, mulching, tender, true, faithful to the earth and her soil. Their nurturing did not disappoint.

The campus was quiet, the grounds around me a verdant masterpiece of summer splendour. I saw one pack of summer-session students huddled together, making a beeline for the cafeteria. But after that, not a soul in sight. I was slowly inching my way across the paths to the library, when, in the blink of an eye, the calm of my internal tranquility was shattered. For some reason, instead of looking ahead a few inches in front of my chair, I looked straight down at the ground below me. There, beneath me, my left foot was poised for its next step. But, at right angles from each of its centers, my laces lay, taut and taunting, on the ground.

My laces. They had come undone.

So did I. My breath caught with a sharp, inward gasp and I didn't dare move. I was terrified of tripping, of falling on the concrete, something unequivocally dangerous for a body like mine. As best as I could with my often uncooperative hands, I clung to the handles on my chair, clutching them in desperation and fear. I was petrified of moving even an inch...the idea of losing my balance and falling unto the hard, unyielding concrete after all I had been through was incomprehensible as well as absolutely terrifying.

"OK, Lord," I prayed, "my sneaker is untied. You know I can't go anywhere. I cannot bend over, much less bend down to the ground, or squat down. I dare not move. Please, please...send me someone."

The campus sat vacant before me and along both sides of me. As to behind me, well, my neck didn't twist well enough to turn around and I could hear no one approaching. So, refusing to give in to the panic rising within me, I talked to the Lord some more.

"You know what I need, Lord and there's nothing else I can do. I'll just try and be still."

Breathe, exhale, drink in grace. Breathe, exhale, drink in grace.

Then, I sensed it - there was someone coming up behind me. I worked my foot and torso around so I could turn my body a bit to the left and then...I saw him. Father Dan. I had always held this particular priest in high esteem and was, truthfully, slightly in awe of him. The work that he had done on a French theologian was something that I, too, wanted to delve into one day. Now, of all possible people on this campus, it was Father Dan who was approaching me. Well, I could never ask *him* to bend down and tie my shoe. To have to ask a student would be embarrassing enough, but Father Dan?

Quickly, I prayed and just as quickly a quip came to my mind. I maneuvered my body forward again and when he had approached my side, I said,

"Father Dan! Good afternoon! How would you like to celebrate Holy Thursday a bit early?" as I looked down at my foot.

For those unfamiliar with our Catholic tradition, we celebrate the

Washing of the Feet during the evening liturgy which begins the Holy Triduum, the three holiest days of the church year: Holy Thursday, Good Friday and The Easter Vigil. This Holy Thursday ritual commemorates Christ showing His disciples His heart of servant leadership. He knelt down at the feet of each disciple present at the meal and washed their dusty, dirty feet.

It has always been a humbling experience for me—to take my shoe and sock off and let a priest wash my foot in front of the whole congregation at Holy Thursday mass.

Fr. Dan got the hint.

Without a moment's hesitation, he said, "Your sneaker is untied!" He knelt down on one knee at my side, put his books to the ground and proceeded to tie my shoe.

I was so deeply touched, so humbled, that this great scholar whom I held in such high esteem, was kneeling down on the hard, hot sidewalk, tying my shoe.

When he had finished his task, he gathered his books and stood up. Once again I felt that familiar feeling of wonderment from watching the complexity of what would be an everyday task for an able-bodied human. Such tasks were inconceivable to anyone in a frozen, paralyzed body. He asked me where I was off to and I said, "The library, but you go ahead. I walk pretty slowly."

"No, no," he said and joined me on the walk there, reassuring me that it was the general direction he was heading in anyway, acting as if he always did a turtle crawl when he was going anywhere on campus.

I asked him what he was teaching and then, with a combined sense of awe and gratitude, I soaked in every word he spoke.

We reached our destinations and parted ways, the eyes of my heart changed forever by the priest who humbly knelt down at my feet to restore my critical and precious sense of safety...and tie my shoelace.

Happy Holy Thursday - in July!

Spirit's words to me

My child, indeed they are my children. I long to feed them too. Love them where they are and keep showing up in your life with your heart open to my presence. The broken ones are waiting for me and don't always know their way back to me. Be the bridge child. Indeed, that was once your calling – building bridges between races at the Y – today build bridges with everyone you meet. Love them with my love, listen with my heart. Go below the surface, hear their pain and fear. You are trying to write on your own. Go easy my child – the book is almost done... Listen a little longer, child, listen to your heart. Yes, you are frustrated now – you want more and are hungry. My child, I know the desires of your heart – I put them there. Be present to me my child, be present today and listen. I have much to reveal to you, much to move in your open heart.

...Come to me with all your worries and concerns child and I will make you whole. I am here, waiting for you, breathing in you. I am here to give you life, direction, meaning and purpose. Your work will reach many, as my hungry souls are everywhere...Come deep within me my child, come deep within. I am your light, your direction and your breath. Yes, your book is done. Work on each piece, I will show you an order and format that will best reach my people, then you will be able to put it into the hands of the editor and publisher, as I have prepared for you. You can go back to school with a new heart, free to embark on a new part of my mission. Indeed it is thundering outside - stay close to me within, stay close to me.

SACRED SPACE

For my priest friends who helped...

It is a phrase our hungry souls
Are instinctively drawn to these days

Sacred space

The souls of this world
Are suffering separation from You
They miss You, Lord
They don't know how to find You
They think they have outgrown You

Sacred space

Hungry souls
As a Eucharistic Minister
at rehab
I see them every week
Traumatized
They lie in a hospital bed or
Sit up in a wheelchair
Wondering
What just happened to them
Through the pain in their eyes
I hear them asking
Where did God go
Are they being punished
Why do they have to hurt so much

What are they going to do now

Sacred space

And their families crowd around their bedsides
Wondering, too
Trying to encourage
To find the right words
Trying to understand this new and surreal reality

Sacred space

And You come
Tiny wafer, round white host
Tiny, powerful presence of hope
You are hope
You come in glory
You come in silence

Sacred space

You know the prayers and pain in each heart
For, as the psalmist tells us
You have created their innermost beings
Sometimes they have strayed from You
You call to them
Your beloved creatures suffering separation from You
You long to have them back

Sacred space

As they receive You in their palms
You feed them in their hearts
Or they receive you on their tongues
Newly able to swallow
Sometimes the tubes in their throats
Keep You away

But not really
You come to their bedside
Longing to feed them
And you still do
Perhaps not physically
Yet
Your presence and peace are there
As You stand within me
Being Eucharist
Bearing Your compassionate, all-embracing blessing
These are Your children
You long to cradle them
Enfold them
Smooth, strengthen
And encourage them
You call them out of their darkness
To the light of your love
It may feel distant to them
And very far away
But You are there

Sacred space

Bless your children Lord
Bless them
They hurt

You are healing
You are wholeness
You are hope
You are
the Sacred Space

Spirit's words to me

My child, breathe deep, be still and listen to me, here in the Adirondack stillness.... My child, listen and be still that I may accomplish great things through you. Be the instrument of my peace and the vessel of my love that I created you for in this time and place. Each day my way will become clear. Indeed, be here and drink in the peace of my words and my mountains, finish my book when you get home, for there are more to come and I have much work for you to do. I know you were frightened and weary of the travel and the bus and your body, oh my child, let me help you. I will make your way clear, as I have with the prophets of old. Seek me and my words and my way will become clear. I want to feed my hungry children, my child, the hunger in you is from me, is my Divine Mercy, my hungry souls, my broken children, yes my child, my heart hurts too. The books will be the beginning. Seek me, I am right here, right here, giving you breath, guiding and directing you, restoring you. Pray for all my children who seek me, for all these wounded souls I have put in your path. Be community with them, be bread - my Body, my Blood I shed for them — to make them whole. Ahh, how I long for them. They are in anguish my child, so many of them, mortal anguish. Breathe, be peaceful, be my vessel and my instrument. I am their health, their grace; you are but the conduit, the earthen, broken vessel. Yes, my child, I have created you in my image MY likeness, I live within you. Live with my love, preach, speak with my love, declare my Word in your quiet presence, preach with words that tell soft and hard stories, laugh, cry, seek me child. I am here to renew you, set you free. Be my peace. Write my child, write.

THE WATCH

It's another cold and damp afternoon. I'm leaning against the equally damp and just as cold cement wall outside of the church. Sometimes it's hard for me to stand for a long time, but I have to be alert for the arrival of the NJ Access Link bus. Since the even-numbered church is on the odd-numbered side of the street, uninitiated drivers tend to miss it. They have to come soon! I'm sore and I'm freezing!

Meanwhile, to keep my mind off of the cold and the damp, I ruminate about the noon Mass. It was quite a liturgical celebration. The opening prayers and scripture readings were beautiful and I always look forward to the homily preached by the young, newly ordained priest from Poland. He somehow manages to make the daily scripture readings apply to my life in a very direct and sometimes humorous, way.

But, no matter what, when it comes time for the congregation to go up to the altar to receive the newly consecrated bread and wine, the Body and Blood of Christ, I'm always more than eager to receive. I think back to the Eucharistic celebration today when I had awkwardly shuffled my way up the main aisle, partially bent over as I often am now. Sitting for any length of time always stiffens me up and standing still for any length of time wearies me. Both slow me down.

I'm feeling weary right now, as I scan the empty street for the bus. I lean back against a damp cement pillar and let my mind wander back to the Mass...

After I had received the host from Father, I turned and limped my way over to the layperson holding the cup of consecrated wine. This was a gentleman I'd seen come in via the side door of the church week after week. He was one of the church's sacristans and whenever I saw him, he reminded me of my late Dad. He was tall and thin (as my Dad was), with a beautiful head of white hair (again, just like Dad's!). Today when this fellow held up the chalice to me and reverently said, "The Blood of Christ," our eyes locked, our souls touched: we became one in Christ. I forgot to breathe during those few seconds of spiritual transformation.

With my fervent "Amen" declaring my spirit of agreement and thanksgiving, I took a sip of the wine and then made my way back to my seat. There I sat down, (kneeling wasn't an option), bowed my head and breathed the breath of heartfelt gratitude for the presence and gift of Jesus within me.

The congregation around me joyfully sang a hymn of adoration (I, of course, had to let them sing for me; sometimes, not being able to sing hurt my heart so much). Then the priest, who had sat down for a few moments to add his voice to the adoration, walked back to the altar and, looking at us with love, blessed us, sending us on our way with the ever familiar exhortation to "Go in the peace of Christ."

It occurs to me now how that peace is my most treasured gift, one that has long eluded me. Yes, I had spent my life feeling *less than*, driven by fears that others would discover how worthless I really felt about myself. But my hospital journey had transformed my heart. I had found peace with the woman God had created me to be.

These reflections bring me a feeling of contentment as I stand in the cold, peering through the mist for the bus. There's still no sign of it. Sometimes it's hard to wait in the dampness and I wish and yearn for a bench to sit upon. Since there is none, I lean into the heavy cement pillar and let my thoughts drift back into the church...

After the Mass had ended and the church started to empty, I still had a few minutes to spare before I needed to go outside to wait for the bus. So, I bowed my head, closed my eyes and went deep into prayer. But then, feeling a movement next to me, I looked up.

It was the man who had given me the Blood of Christ.

He stood by the side of my pew, a total stranger—that is, except for those glimpses I'd had of him over the last few months of my new weekly routine.

He told me his name and said, "and I've been inspired to give this to you."

He reached down into a side pocket of his khaki colored cargo pants and pulled out something on a long silver chain. It was a watch, an old-fashioned pocket watch, much like the ones that men of prominence would tuck inside the vest of their three-piece suits.

As he carefully placed the watch into my hands, I saw that it was encased in silver, with intricate filigree designs swirling around its distinguished, polished face. It was a beautiful piece of artwork.

I stared at it in awe. There was only one person who knew what clocks meant to me.

And that was Jesus.

Clocks were harrowing. *Clocks*...circular standard issue clocks, always high on the wall, always above windows; these were the instruments that marked my bondage within a body that could no longer move. Throughout my long hospital stay, I had spent countless hours staring at the clock on the wall as it mercilessly marked the horrendously slow seconds, the unfathomably long minutes of time dragging its heavy weight through the infinite nights. *Clocks*...faces of white, hands of black, tick, tick, tick, ticking soundless seconds marking the night, mocking my mummified, motionless body.

And, as I laid there, powerless, it taunted me even further, forcing me to remember what I used to be. *What? Can't sleep? An occasional occurrence. Easy to deal with. Say some prayers, roll over on the other side. Still not working? Fling back the covers and go find your study. Write for a little, curl up with a book for a while, until you're nice and tired. Then go back into your room, crawl back under the covers, spouse never even knowing you got up, child nor dog disturbed.*

But that was not my life anymore. Since 'awakening,' sleep came fleetingly, coming only in dribs and drabs. I laid in that hospital bed, totally paralyzed, my body incapable of even the slightest of movements. Always on high alert, my brain pumped adrenaline, cortisol and a host of other neurochemicals through my body, pulsing along with the "food" drip and the antibiotics flowing into the tube in my stomach, or through the PICC line in my arm. Aides came to turn me every two hours so that my immobilized body wouldn't develop bedsores. Despite their greatest efforts to keep their maneuvers as light and as gentle as possible, their slightest touch would engulf my body in flames of pain. In my desperate attempts to hide my misery, I would have to force myself to sing through the excruciating agony of being shifted and moved. Nonetheless, I was grateful for their company since they were my only source of respite from the many lonely hours of the never-ending nights.

And all the while, the minute hand would crawl...literally crawl... showing no mercy throughout the darkness.

My body may have been tirelessly trying to heal, as bodies astonishingly will, but the ticking of that heartless clock denigrated my state of outward stillness, belying the endless turmoil within, mocking me, mocking me... *You can't go anywhere. You can't even move. You are trapped in this night. You are trapped in this bed.* There was nothing, nothing that could offer me mercy from the thousands of passing seconds. But each of those thousands of passing seconds carried with it a thousand desperate, soul consuming, fervid prayers...prayers for me to stay true to You, God, prayers of gratitude for what I did have, prayers for my loved ones, prayers for patients, workers, prayers for so many others.

My very first clock recollection is shrouded...or rather, surrounded by weeks of blackout. But in this memory flash, I am looking at the clock, high up on the hospital wall above the foot of my bed. I remember somehow knowing that it was Confirmation Day in my parish, the day I was supposed to be orchestrating, the culmination of having shepherded the teachers and high schoolers through two years of monthly Sunday morning classes as well as three retreats. This was supposed to be their big day, the one they had worked so hard to get to.

I remember looking at the wall clock and thinking *OK...Sister is in the auditorium now, the corsages have arrived...now she's getting everything coordinated...now she's processing all 120 candidates and their sponsors over to church...*

And interwoven throughout this memory, I also knew that I was in so much pain, that there was some kind of tube in my mouth, in my throat, somewhere, breathing for me. Nonetheless, my mind continued its running commentary, my eyes rigidly focusing on the clock high up on the wall. *OK...10:30...now the Bishop is asking questions...10:50...now he's confirming them.*

And then, all memory once again goes black.

I used to stare at those clocks as they moved ever so slowly, through the long pain-filled nights at rehab and then, through even longer nights at the nursing home. There, time slowed down beyond comprehension, exasperation and fear overtaking me as I was left feeling forsaken and terrified. Even when I was back to the relative safety of rehab again, the clock continued to taunt me, haunt me with its sadistic slowness at night.

And through each languishing movement of that brutal second hand, I did what I had to do: I coped. At the rehab hospital, I "talked" to my siblings in the picture that was propped up on a table to one side of my bed. I knew they were somehow out there cheering for me, that we could do this together...and I prayed for them. I prayed for the intercession of Mother Elizabeth Ann Seton, whose statue I could see on the other side of the bed. She and I became friends then. I knew that she had been a wealthy socialite in lower Manhattan in the late 18th century, but was left widowed and penniless with five children to support. She changed her faith tradition, converting to Catholicism, shocking all who knew her, alienating herself even further from society. I knew that she knew my pain of desperation, of devastation and isolation. I knew that she could teach me to be brave.

And at the nursing home, with no bedside table to hold my treasures, I prayed and talked to my angel friend, Nancy. Nancy had been a friend of mine, a wheelchair user, who had died a few years earlier. She had had spinal cancer in the 80's and had once told me about the nights when she would be screaming in pain since the drugs were not as effective back then. Every night, whenever I glanced at the paper-maché angel that hung from a rod next to my bed, I would think of Nancy, talk to her and ask her to help me.

As the second hand continued to labor its way around and around and around the clock face, I would talk to everyone in heaven and pray... and pray...and pray. The clock's incessant clicking would stop only when the aides came in to turn me every two hours, or clean me when my disconnected, confused body randomly emptied its waste. But the reprieve would be too short-lived. The moment the aides would walk out the door, the cruel and relentless ticking of the seconds on the clock would begin anew, threatening to slowly corrode my sanity as it relaunched its countdown through eternity once again.

But I didn't have a choice. I *had* to hold on.

And so I did. Holding onto my life, my sanity, my prayers, as the minutes on the clock continued...to...simply...crawl.

No. No one knew about the clocks, not one single, breathing human being. Nobody knew anything about the clocks...*nobody but the good Lord Jesus*. And here, cradled in my hands nearly a year later, was the most incredible affirmation I had ever seen. Jesus had told a complete and utter unsuspecting stranger to give me a watch. It was proof, beautiful, ticking, silver encased proof, that He had never left me. He had counted those endless, debilitating and merciless seconds right along with me.

He had never left me alone.

My new friend handed me a business card. He was the COO of a non-profit international foundation with the name of the Blessed Mother Mary in its title. Through a blur of tears, I took the extended card and thanked him. I packed up my things and made my way out of the warm cocoon of the church to await the Access Link bus.

Now here I am, standing, waiting in the cold and damp of my vigil, musing about the gift I had been given.

When the welcomed bus finally arrives, I board, lumbering up the three steps. With a little bit of chit chat, I hand the driver my fare and make my way to my seat. As I click in my seat belt, I think to myself: *I can't wait to get home and pray and meditate about what this watch means.*

But I don't have to wait that long. As soon as my thought finishes, I get a flash of that ridiculous sense of humor that I've come to know so well.

I'm watching you! the familiar voice says, laughing.

In three little words, You, Jesus, give me the watch's meaning:

I'm watching you!

He's taken the most solemn of moments and intentions and entwined it with His silly, wonder-filled, joy-restoring humor.

I crack up in laughter, too.

"You are such a funny boy!" I say, mimicking the tone and words that my late mother would rib at my ever-teasing brother-in-law. I halfway turn to the vacant seat behind me, laughing at myself as I do.

You're watching me!

Spirit's words to me

My child, you are worn out from looking to the past for your fulfillment. Be here with me now – "see I am making all things new." Easy does it my little one. You are scrambling. Be still so that you can hear me. I have not left you alone. Breath and be still. Breathe. I am healing your worn out spirit, renewing your soul. Rejoice in this place of quiet I have called you to, rejoice. You are my child, my little one, can you see as I can see? You're grasping backwards – oh little one, you are lacking trust in me – in a beautiful, full future I have planned for you - where you can write and sing my praise, be in nature, be in my life, my Spirit, feed on my sacramental presence, my liturgy, help the sick and suffering, be my Light.

EUCHARIST

The patients wait for You.
    So many wait for You.
Their faces,
    so filled with anguish.
Their hearts are still raw from their sudden losses,
        the catastrophic changes
            to their lives, their identities, their limbs.
    They are facing each day
        with all the strength and courage they can muster.

And this is where You meet each patient and family member,
    You ache
        to bring them peace amidst their sorrow and uncertainty.
         You meet them
    in the centers of their broken, hungry hearts

In the consecrated bread
        of Your Eucharist
They meet You.
        You bring them comfort
You bring them compassion.

But when I was still a patient
    I didn't know You like that,
        The piece of small, white Eucharistic bread,
    The host, called Holy Communion,
        bearing Your presence, compassion and peace.

Back then, I first received You as a quarter of a host,
　　　at a special Mass in the rehab hospital conference room,
　　　　　two of my priest friends presiding,
　　　　　　　Seton Hall friends gathered to
　　　　　　　　　witness the miracle of transubstantiation.
　　I could hardly swallow,
　　　　it was a skill still new.

The following week I received You in my room,
　　　probably only a small piece of Your host
　　　　　　and I felt this sense of peace afterwards.

It must have been Your presence in the host
　　　　　come to keep my lonely and very bruised heart company.

I received You a few more times
　　　　　but each time the ritual brought only sadness.
　　　　　　　There was no comm-union,
　　　　　　　　　no "in union with"
　　the Eucharistic Ministers
　　　　who would come up to me in my chair,
my big monster of a power chair,
　　　by my bedside
　　　　　　in the late afternoon after therapy.

It seems that somehow I was too intimidating for them,
　　　too frightening in my brokenness.
　　　　　　They must have felt so awkward.
　　They just didn't know what to say.

In retrospect, I wish I could have had the presence of mind
　　to welcome them,
　　　　　put them at ease
　　　　　　　each time they walked up to me,
　　　　　　　　held up the host and said
　　　　　　"Body of Christ,"
　　placed the host on my tongue...

and fled.

No preliminary introduction
        no being-with-me
                no union or fellowship

They fed me Your host and fled.

        I felt so lonely
                they didn't seem to care about me
    to see me inside the broken body.
They forgot that *we* are the Body of Christ,
        each other,
                embodied.

But now You have given me
        the opportunity to bring You to others
                And to be
    Your compassionate Presence

I stand still next to the newly wounded,
    tell them my name and that I've brought You to them.
They are pleased,
    sometimes profoundly overjoyed,
        always grieving.

Then You come to them.
    At first it was startling
            to see the change in their faces.
                Your light
                    when I hold up the sacred bread,
                Your consecrated host.
Their hearts open up to Your food;
    They are Your birds, newly fallen from their nests,
        being fed by You.

You have blessed me profoundly
    allowing me, enabling me to bring You
        to Your hungry
            to Your hurting.

You are the grace that feeds the starving soul
    You are the light that shines amidst the darkness
        You are the hope that renews each weary heart.

Bless Your children at rehab, Lord,
        and at rehab hospitals everywhere.
    Their loss of limb or mobility,
            spinal cord or traumatic brain injuries
    has hurt everyone.

They are all stunned.

Heal their broken hearts, Lord.
    Give them new courage.
        Give them new strength.
            Give them new hope.
    Feed their souls, Lord,
        Feed their souls.

Spirit's words to me

My child, indeed I am here with you. I have freed you. I have promised you I have so much more for you to do. Be dependent on me – you are growing there. The world clamors for your attention - my child, the world needs my food. Come to me, that I may give you food and rest - food and fuel - the deep abiding peace and security of my presence. Oh my child, I love all my little ones, especially my broken ones. With their hearts open, it is easier to find me. Go to them in my peace. That is where your security comes from. I have made you whole in me - your body doesn't matter – I am the truth which guides your heart. Stay open to my immense, inexhaustible grace – grace and compassion. How I long to heal my people, in the dark without me, how frightened and disturbed without me as a rudder for their fragile boats, boats upon the churned-up waters of their lives. They feel lost at sea, abandoned. Go to them with my Eucharist, with my presence. Go to them carrying me in your heart. They will see my love in your eyes. They are so worn and weary - they have been floundering, flailing disturbed, blaming me. Some feel as if their life is at its end - that their misfortune is a cruel joke or punishment – they have nothing to live for - children perhaps, but many feel as if now they have nothing to give them. Oh my child, they need to know that I am here, with them in their hearts. Life's issues and misfortunes may have happened, their hearts and lives torn asunder, but I am here, waiting for them. There is peace in my arms. Comfort, they will find comfort here. In time they will make sense out of their new lives. Oh my child, I long to be their certainty, their compass in there strange and frightening new worlds. Let me be the power they long for, their guide and direction. My children are not being punished - may they gain the grace - it is here, waiting for them – to say yes to me, the still small voice that they are longing for, the presence that I can right their new directions. Oh my child, they need to know how much mercy I have for them, healing mercy. I am not a God who stands in judgment, but one who waits with these open arms to love. Oh my little children, my lost ones, my angry ones, please my child let them know that I wait here for them, their Abba, their healing

Grace, the love they have always longed for - bent or battered in childhood - I am here for them. Criminal, drug dealer - I am here for them. Anxious, broken–hearted young mothers or fathers – I am here for them. Young adults just starting out - I am here for them. Parents of the young adults – heart so wracked in pain at their helplessness for their child – I am here for them. Grandparents, bewildered – I am here for them. Family members feeling guilt and rage and shame – and powerlessness. I am here for them. Single men and women – trying to support families or their own parents – I am here for them. Oh my child, I see their pain. Let them know I hear their cries and pleas. Tell them to be still, I am with them. Their pain will pass - but I will not. They may be struggling with the new or repeated demands of this life, of the demise of their lives as they have known them – but I am a healer of hearts. My grace. Ask them to look for the angels I will send them, for I am there. Some need to renounce their old ways – and my Holy Spirit has the power to heal them and give them strength to ask for new direction, guidance and help. Oh my child, I am here for my sons and daughters – all of them – all races, colors, economic class - street kid, college student, worker, attorney, doctor, nurse, therapist – whatever their role - I am here. I am here to feed them in my healing grace, of love, compassion, forgiveness. My child – let them know how much I love them. Yes, my child these are the final closing words of this book – words of invitation, acceptance and hope. I bring my grace. May each say 'yes' that I may come to strengthen the weak, reorient the lost and bring hope to all, forsaken or afraid - I am with them. I am the peace they thought they would never find, never know again. I am peace. I am grace. Come home to me.

ACKNOWLEDGMENTS

This book is a work of love
by the team we now call
"Hope and Comfort."

Members include:

Dianne Traflet, who planted the seed.

Rich Wolowicz, who endured.

Greg Tobin, for the beginnings.

Kelly Leahy who taught me so much.

Dr. Brian Beyerl,
who not only helped save my life,
but read a prior draft,
and believed in this book.

Pamela Mackey, the other half of my writing group.

Ola Czajkowski
formerly at Paulist Press
who believed and encouraged.

Ellen Weisbord,
for her artistic design.

Cindy Huson,
my patient and efficient
production assistant.

Kaitlyn Quinn, my Seton Hall muse
who joined forces with the
incredibly talented and brilliant
Maggie Kopreski,
and line for line, word for word,
urged me to go deeper
making sure the focus was always on You,
The Spirit of Love.

Thank you all from the bottom of my heart.

ABOUT THE AUTHOR

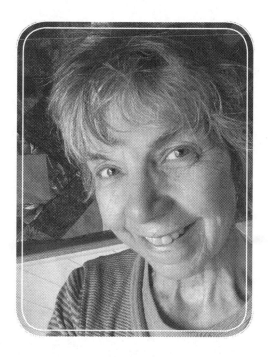

Maryann Hobbie found her life dramatically changed after a traumatic spinal cord injury in the summer of 2013. Her subsequent eight-month hospitalization led her down a pathway of profound physical, emotional and spiritual transformation. Today she lives with PTSD. She is a chaplain, storyteller/speaker and artist who loves all things outdoors. She holds university degrees from Fairleigh Dickinson, Syracuse, Seton Hall, and Drew.

Printed in the United States
by Baker & Taylor Publisher Services